# Animals in Australia

**Malcolm Caulfield**

Vivid Publishing
PO Box 948
Fremantle WA 6959 Australia
vividpublishing.com.au

First published 2018

National Library of Australia Cataloguing-in-Publication entry

Edition: 1st ed.
ISBN:

# Contents

## Acknowledgments

The support, encouragement and criticism of Dr Heather Cambridge was indispensable. Glenys Oogjes, Executive Director of Animals Australia, has been a constant source of inspiration.

My friends and colleagues at the Animal Law Institute provided helpful criticism and comment, and I thank them. They are: Aimee Mundt, Jackson Walkden-Brown, Greta Walker, Susan O'Toole, May Lee, Erin Germantis, Melissa Knoll, Natalie-Anne Morton, Alex O'Brien, Louise Berlicky, Julia Barker, Katie Batty, Hayley Weller, Avishan Bird, Chelsea McPherson, Sophie Harper, Hiana James, Shannen de la Motte, Clair Tighe, Alexandra Geelan, Benny Brown, Kelly Powers and Kate Hewson.

## Foreword

It is now nearly ten years since I wrote the first book on animal cruelty law in Australia.[1] Remarkable things have happened in that time, which have, in my view, altered forever the animal welfare landscape in Australia. Firstly, the horrendous cruelty being inflicted on Australian cattle in Indonesian slaughterhouses was revealed in graphic detail to the Australian public. Determined research by Lyn White of Animals Australia and Bidda Jones of RSPCA Australia culminated in a landmark episode of the ABC's current affairs programme *Four Corners*. Sarah Ferguson, one of Australia's foremost television journalists, was able to present this story in such a way that the upshot was an uprecedented public outcry.[2] Overwhelmed by the response to the programme, the Australian government imposed a temporary suspension of live export of cattle to Indonesia. It also instituted an inquiry led by Bill Farmer (a former ambassador to Indonesia), which in turn resulted in legislative changes aimed at setting standards in overseas abattoirs killing Australian animals.

The second important event was the revelation of widespread and systemic cruelty in the greyhound racing industry in New South Wales, Queensland and Victoria. This second event was similarly analysed and reported in dispassionate detail in another exceptional *Four Corners* investigation. A similar outraged public response resulted. The upshot of this was a number of inquiries, the most notable of which was that carried out by Justice Michael McHugh (formerly of the High Court) in New South Wales.[3] It is the first government inquiry of its kind to expressly acknowledge the need for such animal operations to have a 'social licence' from the wider community. It also acknowledged that 'Australia has been slower to impose [duties of care] on the owners of

---

[1] Caulfield (2008); now available at no charge at https://commons.wikimedia.org/wiki/Main_Page. Search for 'Australian Animal Cruelty Law'.
[2] Jones and Davies (2016)
[3] McHugh (2016)

or those handling animals' than many other jurisdictions. The New South Wales government responded to that report by announcing that greyhound racing in that State would cease from 1 July 2017.[4]

The third remarkable development has been the backlash against these two public reactions to extreme animal cruelty. In the case of both the live export ban and legislative change, and the greyhound racing ban in New South Wales, the relevant industry interests and their political and media supporters mounted a vigorous and effective counter-attack. These counter-attacks have the characteristic of making virtually no mention of the unacceptable cruelty which sparked the bans in the first place; the focus is instead on the economic effects of the ban on those who make money out of the use of the animals concerned. In the case of live export, the farmers, who have always been regarded by the Australian public as holier than the cows they raise and sell, became transmuted into the victims. This prompted politicians from both major parties to come out firmly in support of continuing the live export trade.[5] Some went into the realms of ludicrous hyperbole, saying that live export was essential for Australian agriculture. What they actually meant was that those with vested interests in making money from animals were damned if they were going to be dictated to by animal welfare extremists. In similar vein, the greyhound racing lobby stimulated a huge political outcry, disgracefully supported by the Labor opposition, ultimately forcing the New South Wales government to renege on its commitment to ban greyhound racing.[6] On 19 January 2017, New South Wales Premier Mike Baird resigned, saying he was leaving politics. It has been said that his changed position on the

---

[4] Phillips, C (2016a)

[5] Jones and Davies (2016); A class action has been commenced in the Federal Court, claiming that the then Minister for Agriculture, Joe Ludwig, had no legal justification for implementing the ban: *Brett Cattle Company Pty Ltd v Minister for Agriculture, Fisheries & Forestry* NSD1102/2014 (New South Wales Registry). That case was heard in July 2017 and hearings will continue in September 2018.

[6] Phillips (2016b).

x | F o r e w o r d

greyhound industry ban was instrumental in forcing him from office.[7] This is a tragic outcome, both for former Premier Baird and for the animals. I will not associate myself with those who vilified him as a coward; rather, I think he must be congratulated. It is the people who pressurised him who are deserving of criticism, particularly the Labor Party and Luke Foley, who showed no signs of understanding the moral implications of what they were advocating.

In parallel with this backlash, in 2013 the Liberal/National coalition came to power. Barnaby Joyce was installed as minister with responsibility for agriculture and immediately instituted a policy to disengage the federal government from anything to do with animal welfare.[8]

It therefore appears that, while the Australian public is still not happy with animals being treated badly, there is a substantial sector of the public and more importantly a significant number of politicians in the major parties who are unwilling to translate this concern into action. This is the crucial issue for those concerned with the welfare of animals.

The background against which I write this book is very different from ten years ago. As a result, this book is not primarily a 'law book'. It is a book about the state of animal welfare in Australia; it summarises the landscape of use and abuse of animals in this country, with brief mention of the relevant law where that is appropriate to the narrative. There is greater emphasis on the ethical, economic and political dynamics of the lives of animals in Australia.

The other thing which has happened to me since I wrote the first book is that I have ten years more experience in this area. That experience has included interactions with veterinarians and animal welfare

---

[7] Gerathy, Sarah (2016). *Mike Baird: how NSW Premier went from popular to political scrapheap.* www.abc.net.au/news/2017-01-19/mike-baird-resigns-how-mr-popular-ended-up-on-the-scrapheap/81936
[8] Jones and Davies (2016). Note that as of December 2017 Joyce has given up the Agriculture Portfolio. The Minister is currently David Littleproud.

# Chapter 1    Introduction

The human species is endowed with remarkable intellectual powers. The ability to empathise, feel compassion and derive rules for civilised conduct leads to much that is good. But there is a dark side of aggression, exploitation and cruelty.[9] It is this dark side which must be considered when looking at the plight of the animals who share the world with humans. Professor John Webster can accurately be described as the father of animal welfare science. He has said, 'man has dominion over the animals whether we like it or not'.[10] Humanity can destroy habitats, kill animals for fun, grow and kill them to eat or do experiments on them, ostensibly to benefit the human species. The idea that humans are entitled to exploit non-human animals is described by ethicists Peter Singer and Richard Ryder as 'speciesism'.[11] It is not logical or rational to regard actions benefitting one's own species as necessarily good. One can only suppose that the almost universal acceptance of this concept is a hard-wired evolutionary hangover. This has been described as an 'enormously destructive legacy' as a result of the 'anthropocentric sense of disengagement from the responsibility of preserving our habitat and co-habitants'.[12]

By contrast, there can be a positive interaction between humans and animals and their common environment. Given the ability of humans to analyse their behaviour in a logical fashion, it seems reasonable to expect our species to curb its aggressive, exploitative and cruel instincts. The fact that human beings can appreciate and enjoy beauty support this view.

---

[9] Plato said *'Man is a tame or civilized animal; nevertheless, he requires proper instruction and a fortunate nature, and then of all animals he becomes the most divine and most civilized; but if he be insufficiently or ill-educated he is the most savage of earthly creatures.'*
[10] Webster (2005).
[11] See Chapter 3.
[12] Westbury et al. (2011).

At present, unfortunately, humanity is a long way from achieving this ideal. This is especially so in countries which are less fortunate from the economic point of view. The necessary consequence of the human obsession with economic growth is more extinction of species, more food needed to feed more people, with more animals thereby subjected to cruelty.

It need not be like this. Economics has for many years been obsessed with national output as the measure of progress. This has in turn been used to create and justify inequalities of wealth, coupled with what can only be described as planetary-scale economic vandalism. Modern economics is the ultimate Ponzi scheme, surviving only by increasing the population so those at the top can exploit those at the bottom. It is driven by the unstoppable force of consumerism. However, some economists are now openly saying this model is flawed, and something far more holistic and engaging of individual and planetary maintenance is required.[13] If this view could take hold, it would benefit animals.

At present, concern for animals is not a factor in economic modelling. Economics is concerned with utility of goods or services, and that utility is in turn related to whether or not someone wants to consume those goods and services. Economists struggle with the concept of animal welfare, as it has no utility. And that is where government, made up of those who are charged with the task of making moral decisions, must step in.

This book deals with the landscape in which humans and animals co-exist in Australia. It sets out the history of the interaction and summarises the philosophical and scientific basis of the current position. It contrasts progress of the broad concept of animal welfare with the negative and harmful influence of the increasingly industrial use of animals in modern farming.

---

[13] Raworth (2017).

The book deals briefly with the Australian legislation governing use and abuse of animals. It addresses the regulation of the use of animals and points out how cruelty laws have in the main been undermined by those who use animals for profit or pleasure. It describes the confused state of enforcement of those laws and indicates ways in which the lives of animals could be improved by more enlightened laws and practices.

In Australia, one can observe longstanding views which hold back progress in animal welfare. Sociologist Professor Adrian Franklin explored this phenomenon in detail in his 2007 book *Animal Nation*. He found Australian attitudes to its animals to be uniquely enigmatic. The schizophrenic view of wildlife and introduced species is used by him as a central illustration of the problem. It should come as no surprise that neither of the two major parties in Australia have ever indicated that they intend to make animal welfare a political issue. They avoid these ethical and moral issues. This book is about this seemingly unresolvable tension.

## Chapter 2 Why care?

In perhaps the best known statement about animal welfare, Jeremy Bentham said *'the question is not, 'Can they reason?' nor, 'Can they talk?' but rather, 'Can they suffer?''*. In saying that, Bentham was clearly thinking tacitly that if animals can suffer, then the average human would care about that. Which of course raises the question 'why care?'.

So before going on to consider which animals could possibly suffer, it is important to think about why humans should care about animal suffering.

The answer has to be that humans care because they feel empathy – this is the ability to recognise, understand and share others' feelings.[14] It seems that empathetic responses to images of animal suffering witnessed by human subjects involve activation of the same brain areas as responses to images of human suffering.[15] It has been said that empathy is an appropriate candidate mechanism for altruism, and it appears to be present in several other species.[16] The problem with basing care for animals on the concept of empathy and compassion is that constructing a system of laws based on such ideas is very vexed, as the use of such emotive labels are difficult to define and unify across languages and cultures.[17]

It is part of being a human to feel empathy, concern, compassion, guilt and so on. But the expression of any of those feelings will necessarily be tempered by relevant circumstances. The most important circumstance is the economic position of the observer. Someone who is seriously stressed financially (particularly if they are a farmer, keeping animals) is far less likely to care about the welfare of animals.[18]

---

[14] Wurbel (2009); Urquiza-Haas et al. (2015).
[15] Franklin et al. (2013).
[16] De Waal (2008).
[17] Krech (2016).
[18] Lay and Marchant-Forde (2009).

Of course humans can care about animal suffering, but because they have deeply rooted feelings that humans can use animals for human benefit, there is the inevitable consequence that animal suffering is regarded as less worthy of consideration.[19] Unsurprisingly, the average farmer who uses animals (and by average, I mean one who is not associated with organic or free range farming) is concerned more about welfare aspects which increase productivity, rather than welfare unqualified.[20]

In my view women are more empathetic than men towards animals and so are likelier to want to see an improvement in the conditions of animals. The sociological evidence supports this view. Studies have found that women show stronger affective and weaker utilitarian attitudes towards nonhuman animals than men, a greater concern for animal cruelty issues, less support for exploitation and subordination of animals and a greater concern for animal rights and welfare.[21] Most Australian vegetarians are women and more women than men engage in pro-animal activities.[22] Cornish et al. (2016) reported that female veterinary students were far likelier to be concerned about many aspects of animal welfare.

While there is very good evidence that many people care about animal welfare *per se*, there is also the view that people (and particularly those concerned with law enforcement) should be concerned about animal cruelty because it is often a symptom of other anti-social or criminal behaviour. So, given that it is very likely that the reason we care comes from our ability to empathise, it is perhaps not surprising that studies of those who commit acts of animal cruelty have found that a high

---

[19] Gullone (2012).
[20] Cornish et al. (2016).
[21] Herzog (2007); Phillips et al. (2011); Urquiza-Haas et al. (2015).
[22] Chen (2012).

proportion of perpetrators have what psychologists call the 'Callous-Unemotional' trait.[23]

Phil Arkow rightly points out that depicting animal abuse as a human welfare concern is one way to make progress with those in power, such as policy makers, law enforcers and the like.[24] There is considerable evidence that those who are cruel to animals also have a propensity for violence towards humans. Cruelty to animals can be said to be deviant; however, the study of this issue is clouded by public acceptance of certain behaviours, which are ostensibly cruel, as acceptable.[25]

Moreover, just because cruelty to animals is regarded as deviant, and thereby might be made illegal, it does not mean to say cruelty to animals is regarded in as serious a way as illegal and cruel behaviour towards humans. The opposite is true, in that illegal cruelty to animals is held to be on a much lesser scale.[26]

Mild and isolated forms of animal cruelty may be part of normal exploratory behavior during childhood. Poor parental behaviour can be instrumental in the development of tendencies for children to be cruel to animals.[27] Although many of those who are cruel to animals are motivated by 'fun', there are many other motivations for the behaviour.[28]

Another strong indication that society regards cruelty to animals as behaviour outside the acceptable norm is its inclusion in diagnostic

---

[23] see Gullone (2012).
[24] Arkow (2012).
[25] Gullone (2012) gives examples including practices engaged in during rodeos; one could also include the routine surgical mutilations of farm animals without pain relief, routine brutal treatment of farm animals, and the inevitable cruelty associated with hunting.
[26] Gullone (2012).
[27] Gullone (2012).
[28] Gullone (2012).

criteria for Conduct Disorder in the US *Diagnostic and Statistical Manual of Mental Disorders.*[29]

The two theoretical models of animal cruelty are that animal cruelty in childhood is predictive of later violence towards humans ('the Violence Graduation Hypothesis'), and the Deviance Generalization Hypothesis, which suggests that animal cruelty co-occurs with aggressive and anti-social behaviour in general.[30] The first of these has been criticised as being based heavily on self-reporting recollections of people in penal institutions.[31]

In Australia, Gullone has provided evidence showing that those charged with animal cruelty offences are more than 3 times as likely as other offenders to also be charged with offences against the person. This provides further (local) support for the idea that animal cruelty occurs along with other antisocial behaviours or acts of violence against people.[32] Both serial killers and mass murderers have been found to have a previous history of violence towards animals.[33] There is a very strong correlation between perpetrators of domestic violence and cruelty to animals; in particular abusive partners (men) will often threaten the other partner's pet with violence.[34]

Another consideration which is involved in motivating people to be concerned about animal welfare is that concern for animal welfare is often, at least in the mind of the consumer, associated with concern about food safety and quality.[35]

---

[29] see Gullone (2012).

[30] Gullone (2012).

[31] Beirne, P. (2004). From animal abuse to interhuman violence? A critical review of the progression thesis. *Society & Animals* 12, 39-65.

[32] see Gullone (2012).

[33] Gullone (2012),.

[34] Volant, AM et al. (2008). The relationship between domestic violence and animal abuse: an Australian study. *Journal of Interpersonal Violence* 23, 1277-1295.

[35] Vapnek and Chapman (2010).

The conclusion is that humans do care about animals in a way that is not entirely selfish and is based on the human-animal similarity. I don't think it is something which can be described as advantageous to the human species in the Darwinian, evolutionary sense; the fact it is real and significant is all that matters. But there is still the prevailing instinct (and I think it is an instinct) to regard care for other humans as somehow more worthy than care for animals.

# Chapter 3   Ethics, morals and politics

## Animals, philosophy, religion and science

### Early philosophers

The Western attitude to animals has its roots in Judaism and Greek philosophy. These roots became united in Christian precepts.[36]

Greek philosophy included consideration of the human-animal relationship. Pythagoras (570-495 BC) believed that animals and humans have souls, which can be reincarnated. His was not a widely accepted position.

By contrast, the views of Aristotle (384-322 BC), which reflected the concept that the human species was intrinsically superior to the rest of the animal kingdom, became widely influential for many centuries (indeed, millenia). Thus, says Aristotle, animals are created for the sake of man, and humans govern animals.

This was certainly the position of Judeo-Christian religious teaching. Genesis (1:26-28) expressly refers to the dominion of man, made in God's image, over all creatures. St Thomas Aquinas (1225-1274) reiterated the position espoused by Aristotle, casting it in the same way as the biblical pronouncements. He was also of the opinion that animals were 'devoid of the life of reason', being moved 'by a kind of natural impulse'. Being 'irrational', they had no fellowship with man 'in the rational life', and divinity did not extend to them. That lack of fellowship with humans thereby gave humans complete dominance over animals, including the right to kill them, presumably without feeling bad about it.

Again echoing Aristotle, Aquinas developed the theme that cruelty to animals was a bad thing, but only because people who were cruel to

---

[36] Singer (1975).

animals had a tendency to behave cruelly to other people.[37] Many Western philosophers adopted this view. Both Kant and John Locke talked about 'hardening of the heart' in those who were cruel to animals.[38] Kant (1724-1804) reflected the views of Aquinas when he said that animals could not be moral agents because they 'do not experience themselves'; they were thereby not owed any duties.

Descartes (1596-1650) expanded on the idea of animals lacking a soul, and thereby lacking reason. In his opinion, only humans could communicate through language; animals were restricted to 'natural or instinctive signs'. This drew him to the conclusion that animals were no different from machines. In the following century Rousseau (1712-1785) expressed similar sentiments seeing nothing in any animal but 'an ingenious machine'. The critical distinction between animals and humans was that the latter had free will, whereas the former 'respond by instinct'.

The Scottish philosopher David Hume (1711-1776) broke with these views. He saw that humans performed actions 'which tend to self-preservation, to obtaining pleasure and avoiding pain'. This was also the case with other creatures, such that 'all our principles of reason and probability carry us with an invincible force to believe the existence of a like cause'. This sort of view was very much the exception to the prevailing attitudes. Irish-born philosopher Francis Hutcheson (1694-1746) was another ahead of his time on human treatment of animals, and theologian Humphrey Primatt (c. 1742), in his groundbreaking treatise *A Dissertation on the Duty of Mercy and the Sin of Cruelty to Brute Animals*, likewise advanced a convincing argument that it was wrong to inflict pain on animals. [39]

---

[37] see Rollin (1992).
[38] Quoted in Gullone (2012).
[39] See Garrett (2007).

So as the eighteenth century drew to a close, there were big changes afoot, including views in (higher) society about treatment of animals. Given the social structure of the time, compassion towards animals was clothed in a sub-plot of concern about the behaviour of the unwashed rabble. But this was all part of the wider emerging awareness and involvement in political issues of the middle and upper classes.[40] Slavery was under attack and the French were openly talking about issues of equality amongst people. Jeremy Bentham was an English philosopher who achieved much in his life. He set the scene for a rational basis for caring about animals, in a fashion which is recognisable today in many respects. In *An Introduction to the Principles of Morals and Legislation* (1789) he said:

> '*What other agents then are there, which, at the same time that they are under the influence of man's direction, are susceptible of happiness? They are of two sorts: (1) other human beings who are styled persons, (2) other animals, which on account of their interests having been neglected by the insensibility of the ancient jurists, stand degraded into the class of things...If the being eaten were all, there is very good reason why we should be suffered to eat such of them as we like to eat: we are the better for it, and they are never the worse. They have none of those long protracted anticipations of future misery which we have...If the being killed were all, there is very good reason why we should be suffered to kill such as molest us; we should be the worse for their living, and they are never the worse for being dead. But is there any reason why we should be suffered to torment them? Not any that I can see. Are there any why we should not be suffered to torment them? Yes several. The day has been, I grieve to say in many places it is not yet past, in which the greater part of the species, under the denomination of slaves, have been treated by the law exactly upon the same footing, as, in England for example, the inferior races of animals*

---

[40] Kean (1998).

*are still. The day may come, when the rest of the animal creation may acquire those rights which never could have been withholden from them but by the hand of tyranny. The French have already discovered that the blackness of the skin is no reason why a human being should be abandoned without redress to the caprice of a tormentor. It may come one day to be recognized, that the number of the legs, the villosity of the skin, or the termination of the os sacrum, are reasons equally insufficient for abandoning a sensitive being to the fate? What else is it that should trace the insuperable line? Is it the faculty of reason, or perhaps, the faculty of discourse? But a full-grown horse or dog, is beyond comparison a more rational, as well as a more conversable animal, than an infant of a day, or a week, or even a month, old. But suppose the case were otherwise, what would it avail? The question is not, Can they reason? nor, Can they talk? but, Can they suffer?'.*

## Religion

Many people would say that there is no point arguing about morality, because it is God-given.[41] But one cannot deny that down the ages religions have had a great influence in defining moral codes.[42] And if those codes are good, it hardly matters whether they have been made by God or people.

The Old Testament is very clear about the dominance of Man ('made in God's image'), being given dominion over all the creatures of the Earth, although there are a few mentions which could be viewed as reflecting a 'stewardship', rather than a 'dominion' view.[43]

While more modern Christians might want to elide the love of Christ with love of animals, the New Testament is devoid of any such mention.

---

[41] Broom (2006).
[42] Broom (2006).
[43] Singer (1975).

The driving forces of theological thought in early Christianity were unequivocal in their view that (for example) while it was forbidden to kill other human beings (but of course even that view was tempered by practicalities, such as wars, or dealing with heretics), it was permissible to kill 'irrational animals'. Saint Augustine (354-430 AD) said this view was justified because animals had no reason, plus of course the Creator permitted it.

In religions of the Indus Valley Civilization, the belief that ancestors return in animal form led to the view that animals should be treated with the respect given to humans. This belief is exemplified in Jainism. The Indian emperor Ashoka (274-232 BC) forbade killing living things for food or for sacrifice. Buddhists believe that it is a sin to kill any living thing.[44] The position of Islam is that to treat animals badly is to disobey the will of Allah. Muhammad taught that animals should only be killed out of necessity.

While one may be cynical about religion, it is true nevertheless that many religious people have spoken out eloquently on behalf of animals. Hilda Kean (1998) provides the example of John Wesley, founder of Methodism, who made it clear that animal cruelty was unacceptable.

The problem for believers in religion (and therefore a God) is that there has to be at least a very real possibility that God (any god) is a figment of the human imagination, and religion is in fact just a political tool by which one group manipulates another. That said, it is hardly surprising that the harsh reality for animals in the world today is they get little relief from religious tenets. Indeed, there is evidence that there is a negative correlation between religiosity and concern for farm animal welfare.[45] This is entirely consistent with adherence to religious tenets being essentially human-centred.

---

[44] Szucs et al. (2012).
[45] Cornish et al. (2016).

Another powerful force which, like religion, does not rely on logic or reason in its propositions concerning animals, is tradition or culture. Paula Casal (2003) has given graphic accounts of practices in Spain, justified in the name of religion, which are truly blood-curdling. She has also referred to the cynical move by Spanish politicians to avoid a European Union ban on bullfighting on the basis it was a traditional activity. Traditional practices are used as justification for all sorts of cruel activity, such as whaling.

## Science

The work of Charles Darwin in the middle of the nineteenth century revolutionised the relationship between the human species and animals. The idea that humans were descended from animals by evolution directly challenged the concept of the supremacy of the human species. As Darwin said 'man in his arrogance thinks himself a great work, worthy of the intervention of a deity. More humble and, I believe, true to consider him created from animals'. Although Darwin did not have the tools of modern science at his disposal, he was obviously a keen and insightful observer of the world and its inhabitants. He felt there was 'no fundamental difference between man and the higher animals in their mental faculties' and that 'the lower animals, like man, manifestly feel pleasure and pain, happiness and misery'. Having said that, Peter Singer points out that Darwin did not expressly make the link between evolution from animals and the human species until 1871, with the publication of *The Descent of Man*.[46]

---

[46] Singer (1975).

At this point it is useful to jump ahead to modern knowledge and briefly set out a simplistic view of how living things have evolved. [47]

| Organisms | Last common ancestor (millions of years) |
|---|---|
| Chimpanzee | 8 |
| Macaque | 25 |
| Rodent | 75 |
| Marsupial | 140 |
| Reptiles and birds | 310 |
| Amphibians | 340 |
| Fish | 440 |
| Sea squirts | 565 |
| Starfish etc | 570 |
| Jellyfish | 590 |
| Sponges | 800 |
| Fungi | 1100 |
| Plants | 1200 |

It is clear that the fundamental biology of even early animals is the same as human beings. All animals use nucleic acid (DNA, RNA) to encode their proteins, and reproduce, they use the same sort of metabolism (making the high energy molecule ATP, which is the 'fuel' of cells), and they use enzymes to drive metabolic processes.

The discovery of the structure of DNA by Watson, Crick, Wilkins and Franklin, which was published in 1953, set the stage for the amazing advances of the last few decades. Because knowledge of the DNA sequence of a gene could reveal which proteins were encoded by the gene, the ability to sequence DNA enabled the gathering of information about how cells of different species worked. The Human Genome Project represented a pinnacle of achievement, and indicated the extent of similarities between human beings and other animals. The

---

[47] Kirkwood (2006).

concept that humans are intrinsically different from animals has therefore been finally rebutted. Given the enormous increase in understanding of both human and animal biology, it is increasingly difficult to justify treating humans and animals differently.

## Ethics and morals

Ethics is the study of moral issues. Something is moral if it relates to whether something is right or wrong.[48] Moral principles are the body of obligations and duties that a particular society requires of its members.[49] Of course if one doesn't believe in a God setting down what is 'right' and 'wrong', one has to decide for oneself.

Many would take the view that there is no need for academic debates about the position of animals in modern society. After all, everybody knows that cruelty is wrong, and it's as simple as that. Or is it? As you start to consider the way animals have been regarded, and where we are today, it is apparent that views concerning animals have changed dramatically and are still changing. It is necessary, therefore, to consider the current perception of animals and to ask hard questions about how much we are justified in exploiting animals, and how much we owe them.

A key question is whether animals have value and if so, what kind of value. That question is in turn dependent on how one views the idea of humans having dominion and power over animals. If that means animals only exist to benefit humans, then the value of the animal will be determined according to the level of that benefit and its welfare will only have significance as it affects human use. However, if the concept of 'dominion' over animals extends to including 'stewardship' and an obligation to care for animals, then it is realistic to regard each animal as having intrinsic value.[50] There are arguments that this may involve

---

[48] Broom (2006).
[49] Szucs et al. (2012).
[50] Broom (2014).

having respect for the 'dignity' of an animal. Nussbaum has suggested institutions and individuals have a duty to protect and promote the flourishing of an individual's capabilities. Thus, she says this approach is animated by an Aristotelian view that complex natural organisms are worthy of awe; it is therefore sensible to accord respect to animals and recognize their dignity.[51] Interestingly, this concept of respect is repeated many times in the National Health and Medical Research Council's Code dealing with use and care of animals in relation to scientific experiments (see Chapter 8).

Concepts about which individuals should be the subject of moral actions ('moral agents') have changed with improved communication and increasing knowledge of the functioning of animals and humans. Living things that are thought to experience emotions, including the capacity to feel pleasure and pain, are more likely to be attributed moral rights.[52] People are more likely to refrain from causing harm if those in their social group may come to know about what they have done. Today, information about what someone has done can literally be promulgated worldwide almost instantly.[53]

Recognising an animal as qualifying as the subject of moral actions immediately raises the issue of sentience. Widespread acceptance of studies demonstrating the intelligence and cognitive abilities of members of other species has encouraged the expansion of the range of species which can be the subject of moral actions.[54] However, Broom (2011) points out that all animals are not equal in this regard, even when they are the same animals. He refers to the different treatment a rabbit will receive depending on whether it is a pet, an experimental subject in a laboratory, an animal grown for food, or a feral creature in the wild which eats farmers' crops and digs holes.

---

[51] Nussbaum (2006).
[52] Urquiz-Haas et al. (2015).
[53] Broom (2003).
[54] Broom (2011).

It is true that animal interests are denigrated as less worthy than human needs.[55] While survey data shows that significant numbers of Australians state that they support human-equivalent rights for animals, those same people are completely inconsistent in their view of different classes of animals. Most notably, animals grown and killed to provide meat are attributed fewer rights, while companion animals are regarded as having more rights.[56]

Influenced by religion, the prevailing view to this day is that humans are superior, rational beings, at the top of an evolutionary pyramid. This gives them the right to use animals to suit their own ends. Bertrand Russell (1872-1970) identified the logical fallacy several decades earlier when he said: 'there is no impersonal reason for regarding the interests of human beings as more important than those of animals. We can destroy animals more easily than they can destroy us; that is the only solid basis of our claim to superiority'. It is the 'arbitrary favouring of one species' interests over another'. This is speciesism, a logical extension of an anthropocentric world view.[57] More recently, eminent evolutionary biologist Richard Dawkins has put all this into perspective, noting that humanity is put 'on a pedestal miles higher than the surrounding territory' and (with his trademark bluntness) 'a human foetus that has approximately the anatomy and brainpower of a worm is accorded more status than an adult chimpanzee' and goes on to remark that chimpanzees have more rights than cows. He compares lack of compassion for animals with the views of ordinary people in Nazi Germany, describing this as a kind of laziness; at the most people are vaguely uneasy, but justify their lack of concern by the thought 'everyone else is doing it'.[58]

---

[55] Arkow (2012).

[56] Chen (2016).

[57] Ryder (1989).

[58] Tom Whipple (13 May 2017) *Richard Dawkins: 'When I see cattle lorries, I think of the railway wagons to Auschwitz'*. The Times.

Some have posited that speciesism is positively associated with 'ethnic outgroup attitudes'. In other words, those who are prejudiced towards others on an ethnic basis are very likely to be speciesist, and also to perceive vegetarianism as a threat.[59]

Peter Singer is a prominent philosopher and ethicist whose book *Animal Liberation*, published in 1975, transformed thinking on the position of animals in society. He eloquently criticised the common approach to treatment of animals, which is based on speciesism. This conclusion is set out in the first chapter of the book, *All animals are equal*. Singer is a utilitarian, so echoes the view of 19th century philosopher J.S. Mill that the 'right' action or policy is that which will result in the maximum utility; that is, the expected balance of satisfaction versus dissatisfaction, in all sentient beings affected by the action or policy. Highly-regarded animal welfare lawyer Alex Bruce has highlighted the fact that, in reality, all utilitarian philosophies are effectively contaminated by an anthropocentric underlay, such that human views will always be preferred when there is a conflict between the interests of animals and the interests of humans.

Influential animal welfare scientist Donald Broom[60] suggests that taking the utilitarian approach to animal welfare may be incomplete. Striking the balance on the basis of the average or overall good of collections of all the sentient individuals affected does not take account of an important point. This is that humans (and indeed other animals) interact with and have concerns for other individual beings. Thus, moral codes are framed to consider effects on individuals as well as populations of individuals. Broom and Fraser (2007) illustrate this by reference to the example of an individual causing damage to many others. Many persons would take the view that this does not justify extreme action against the individual – the obvious example is imposing the death penalty. The inference is that some rights or principles take precedence over a

---

[59] Dhont et al. (2016).
[60] Broom (2003).

strictly utilitarian analysis. Having said that, all rights must be tempered with regard to the potential damage which can be caused to others if those rights can be exercised in all circumstances. In Broom's view, arguments based on obligations achieve better results than seeking to assert rights.[61]

The ethical concern was summarised by Peter Singer, giving evidence to the Australian Senate Committee on Animal Welfare in 1989:

> *'I think what you should really be asking for the purposes of investigation of intensive farming is: 'is this at all a tolerable life for the animals, looking at the life as a whole?'. I believe that if you look at the cases of intensive farming and a life that basically consists of a year to eighteen months being crowded into a battery cage and then getting thrown out and killed, or in the case of a breeding sow, say months on end spent unable to walk around, turn around, socialising in the normal way, simply lying there with nothing to do, then I think that it is pretty clear that that is not a tolerable life for an animal. I think that minimum standards ought to be implemented to make sure that they can have for the duration something that we can regard as a reasonable life to inflict on another creature.'*

At this point, it is important to note that some commentators have contrasted two positions regarding the treatment of animals. The first position has been described as 'welfarist'.[62] This designation reflects the idea that people can exploit animals, including killing and eating them, provided the animals are treated 'humanely' and not inflicted with 'unnecessary suffering'. It involves working to achieve incremental improvements in the lot of animals. Richard Haynes (2011) has argued that this welfarist concept originated with the foundation in 1926 of the University of London Animal Welfare Society. The term 'welfarist' and

---

[61] Broom (2003); (2014).
[62] See Bruce (2012).

its use in the definition of animal welfare by some commentators serves to create confusion. This is because the term 'animal welfare' now has a scientific meaning which is different.

The second position is that of 'animal rights'. The view of animal rightists is that the welfarist approach should be rejected in favour of a much more extreme position. The rightist view is that animals can not be exploited in any way. Many would regard this position as fanciful; John Webster has described this as striving for the attainment of 'Eden'.[63] What the 'welfarist' view does accept, and the 'rights' view does not, is that in the real world it is likely that for some considerable time, most people would regard it as entirely reasonable to exploit animals.

To understand the animal rightists' position, one has to first consider what a 'right' is. The law would regard a right as a valid moral claim that society says must always be respected (different then, to an 'interest').[64] However, even that causes problems. Rights are created by people (and expressed in the law). So they can never be absolute, because the law can qualify anything. It can define 'black' to include 'white'. So are there 'natural rights'? Not according to Jeremy Bentham, who described natural rights as 'nonsense upon stilts'. This is in essence because an absolute right cannot be checked in any way; anarchy is the result.[65]

Rights do not pop into existence out of a vacuum; they are granted by humans and are in that sense a completely artificial construct. Modern legal theorist Rawls has been influential in developing a theory of how rights work.[66] He suggested a 'contractarian' view of society whereby members of society in essence agree to be bound by rules governing the way society works. This can only work for 'rational beings' who

---

[63] Webster (2005).

[64] Bruce (2012).

[65] see the entry in the *Internet Encyclopedia of Philosophy* at www.eip.utm.edu/bentham.

[66] see Abbey (2007).

understand the reciprocal basis of this social contract. So animals, which cannot have any understanding of a contract, are excluded by definition from this theory of justice. But then according to this logic, so are infants and brain-damaged or mentally impaired people. This just doesn't make sense.[67] As Garner puts it,[68] applying this sort of logic, the conclusion is that the state must remain neutral when it comes to competing conceptions of the moral status of animals. However, Abbey has pointed out that Rawls himself acknowledged that his theory of justice as fairness failed to encompass all moral relationships, essentially being restricted to inter-human relationships.[69] Regardless of these rather theoretical considerations, there is in fact nothing to stop lawmakers from giving animals as many rights as they want.

The views of animal rights advocate Tom Regan illustrate the rightist position.[70] He believes animals should not be used in science, should not be grown and killed to be eaten and should not be used for 'sport'. He is not prepared to accept that things can be improved for animals by more humane treatment. One of his core points is that animals have inherent value; they are all 'experiencing subjects of a life' and so have the right to be treated properly. They are 'moral patients' which are owed duties. Legal theorist Gary Francione goes even further. He is unprepared to accept that animal suffering, or animal death is any different from human suffering or human death. He rejects the concept that humans should have total and unconstrained power over animals.

## Animals as property

At present, the legal classification of animals as property reflects the widely held belief that animals are commodities and that it is reasonable to exploit them. Many animal advocates and scholars of animal law have concentrated heavily on this property construct. They

---

[67] Rollin (1992).

[68] Garner (2002).

[69] Abbey (2007).

[70] eg Regan (1987).

maintain that equal consideration of animal and human interests cannot be achieved while animals are regarded as property. This is probably so if one accepts Blackstone's definition of property from a legal point of view – 'the sole and despotic dominion which one man claims and exercises over the external things of the world, in total exclusion of the right of any other individual'.[71] This really is the Englishman's castle view of the world.

Francione vigorously espouses the view that animals will never be treated properly while they are regarded as property.[72] I agree with Garner's analysis that this argument is flawed.[73] Removal of the property status of animals will not guarantee anything, let alone proper treatment of animals. Stating the obvious, wild animals are not the property of anybody, but they suffer nevertheless from the depredations of humans. Abolishing the property status of animals and giving them 'rights' may also be meaningless, in the absence of proper enforcement of those 'rights'. The parallels with human 'rights' are obvious. In other words, this sort of debate is sterile; the only thing which will improve the lot of animals is a real change in the attitudes of society. In any case, the 'property' classification is not inconsistent with proper treatment of animals. We are a long way beyond the idea that the rights of an owner regarding his or her property are absolute. It is therefore apparent that obligations can be imposed on the owner of an animal. Furthermore, the argument that animals cannot protect themselves while they are regarded as property is a false argument, as society is quite able to act to protect the otherwise helpless, including the very young and the mentally incapable. There is no reason why protection of the welfare of animals cannot be achieved successfully by government entities, regardless of whether animals are property or not.

---

[71] See William Blackstone (1763), 'Commentaries on the Laws of England', https://ebooks.adelaide.edu.au/b/blackstone/william/comment/book2.1.html

[72] see Francione (1995); (2000).

[73] Garner (2002).

Changing the semantics around the descriptor of animals as property will not be a magic bullet.[74] Likewise, granting animals 'rights' will achieve nothing, unless any such change happens as a consequence of a change in attitudes.[75] The change in attitudes has to come first. And frankly, the views of Regan, Francione and others are baffling to most people. When animal movements demand too much, in the words of John Webster, they achieve little.[76] It is all very well to want perfection, and to want it now, but this flies in the face of reality. The overall balance is that progress is being made, albeit slowly. Progress can be expected to result from a gradual improvement of living standards certainly in the West, and progressively more elsewhere. Webster has remarked that 'man's humanity or inhumanity to man and other animals tends to vary in direct proportion to his own comfort, wealth and security. It is easier to care for others when one's own survival is not under threat'.[77] This is, in my view, a key point. Moreover, fixating on 'animal rights' can end up with people 'trapped in their seductive web...unwilling to roll up our sleeves and set to work helping animals the hard way'. So said Jonathan Lovvorn, a highly experienced and effective animal lawyer and academic in the USA.

### 'Welfarism' *versus* 'rightist' – a personal view

Regarding all the various ethical viewpoints, ranging from the 'welfarist' to the 'rightist' and all points in between, in my view the most influential works have been those of Peter Singer. Their power lies in their clear and logical expression which are vividly illustrated by reference to what actually goes on with animals used by humans. He has a unique ability

---

[74] Bruce (2012) refers to Sunstein's point that Francione has not demonstrated that the property status of animals is inconsistent with recognising their value.

[75] Posner (see Bruce, 2012) has noted that the 'rightist' argument suffers from not actually being able to define what rights should be assigned to non-human animals.

[76] Webster (2005).

[77] Webster (2005).

to point out the glaring inconsistencies between what we say we would like to happen, and what we actually do.

Alex Bruce (2012) neatly summarised it when he said '...the point of exploring these philosophical approaches to animal welfare is not to construct abstract and empty theories. Nor is the point to construct complicated theories that make it difficult, if not impossible, for people to understand what is being said'. Similarly, animal welfare scientist David Fraser (2012) has suggested that an alternative approach to a theory-based approach is to use 'care-based' ethics, by application of 'virtues such as care and empathy'. He espouses providing good lives for animals in our care, treating suffering with compassion, trying to be aware of unseen harm, and avoiding upsetting balances of nature in a way that compromises animals.

Perhaps a sensible ethical framework, which can be turned into sensible laws, is to use a 'guardianship' model, as first proposed by Joyce Tischler (1977). This makes sense, because it resonates with the situation of other beings which society looks after in that way, because they cannot look after themselves; very young children and intellectually disabled persons are obvious examples.

Finally, as lawyer Mike Radford says, it is absolutely the case that the truth about how we should treat animals, and therefore the laws which set those limits or impose the duties is not self-evident. The law must reflect a moral consensus, otherwise it will be impossible to enforce, and will be worse than useless. However 'a law which is ahead of its time has [often] had the effect of educating the public eventually to endorse the policy it represents'.[78] Perhaps the best approach, as Don Broom has suggested, is for humans to learn to respect all animal life, with all that follows.[79]

---

[78] Radford (2001).
[79] Broom (2014). See also Alex Bruce's quotes regarding the thoughts of Albert Schweitzer on this subject (Bruce 2012).

## Politics

In my view, the most powerful force which influences political decisions regarding the plight of animals in Australia is the farming lobby. This consists of not just the farmers themselves, but their representative bodies, such as the National Farmers Federation, and bodies representing particular types of animal enterprises, such as Australian Pork Limited. The power of the farmers and of these bodies is enhanced by the high regard that the majority of Australians have for farmers.[80] There are many surveys confirming this view, including those conducted by farming bodies.[81]

My personal opinion is that the farming lobby has influence and power which is disproportionately large, given its contribution to the national economy. Farm production in 2015-16 was worth about $31 billion dollars, representing roughly 1.9% of gross domestic product.[82] The agricultural sector in that period employed 282,000 people, roughly 2.4% of employed persons. In 2013-14, the agriculture and fishing sector paid $563m in taxation, representing about 0.17% of the Australian Taxation Office's tax receipts.[83]

On the other side of the balance sheet, agriculture uses just over 50% of Australia's land, a total of 385 million hectares.[84] It is difficult to enumerate the benefits and concessions which farmers receive from taxation authorities. These include the ability to average income over years, offsetting losses against income from other sources, transfer of property within families without incurring 'stamp duty' liability, diesel fuel rebate and deferral of income tax using the farm management

---

[80] see Parbery and Wilkinson (2012).

[81] Chen (2016).

[82] ABARES (2015).

[83] Australian Taxation Office Taxation statistics 2013-2014, All tax returns. www.ato.gov.au/About-ATA/Research-and-statistics/in-detail/Taxation-statistics/Taxation-statistics-2013-2014.

[84] ABARES (2015); Geoscience Australia www.ga.gov.au/scientific-topics/national-location-information-dimensions.

deposits scheme.[85] Many current farming practices damage the environment and are a source of greenhouse gases.[86]

The National Party is the 'Farmer's Party'. Former Liberal Party leader John Hewson recently had this to say about the Nationals:

> *'The National Party has always been less pure than conservatives on key economic issues. Issues such as free trade – wanting free access to foreign markets..., while seeking to simultaneously impose health, quarantine and anti-dumping restrictions on foreign competitors they may face in our domestic economy, and also demanding various subsidies and support for farmers...diesel rebates, concessional loans and other subsidies. Similarly on welfare – the Nats are hard on the disadvantaged, unless they are farmers facing drought, flood and fire.'*[87]

Given the small contribution of the farming industry to national wealth, taxpayers are nevertheless willing to give financial support to farmers affected by droughts, floods, depression and every other problem they are faced with. Moreover the predominantly city-dwelling taxpayers are also expected to cheerfully endure a sustained flow of insults from farmers' representatives. The farming bodies relentlessly paint farmers as superior to the ignorant city slickers. Don Watson got it right when he said *'So long as the people of the country are the real Australians, other people are less real..this might be only to say less distinctively Australian...then again it might mean effete, parasitic bludgers: sybarites, late risers, people with no conception of what it is to be at the mercy of the elements'*.[88] To illustrate, after the revelations of

---

[85] H&R Block (2016) *Farmers! Harvest a great outcome with H&R Block.* www.hrblock.com.au/tax-tips/farmers-harvest-a-great-outcome-with-h-and-r-block.
[86] Garnett et al. (2013).
[87] Beware the 'new conservatives' motivated by ambition and ego. *The Age* 5 January 2017.
[88] Watson (2014).

horrendous cruelty in the greyhound industry and New South Wales Premier Mike Baird's brave attempt to ban greyhound racing, one of the farming MP's said Baird's decision was '...one pitched at latte-sipping keyboard warriors, long sock-wearing elitists from the North Shore, who see life through rose-coloured glasses...'.

Why do the city-dwelling taxpayers put up with this opprobrium? Again, Watson suggests the answer: *'That the great majority of Australians live in cities does not diminish the power of the bush, but on the contrary adds an exotic or romantic dimension to the suburban cliché of our existence. The bush is where the real Australians live, and whatever hurts or threatens them the rest of the country feels...'.* Politicians exploit this fondness for all things 'bush', wearing identifiable 'bush' headgear and waxing lyrical on concepts like 'mateship'.[89] Self-evidently, this is nonsense: *'Australian farming is ...an ideology as self-justifying, exclusive and delusional as the doctrine of God-given right under which the land was first appropriated. It is a story...of human beings granting themselves an option over all creation, to be exercised at will and accordance with any whim or impulse...'.*[90]

Of course the farming lobby's influence increases when a Liberal – National coalition government is in power. In the 2016 Federal election, the Coalition won a total of 76 seats. The Labor party won 69 seats, a difference of 7 seats, and there were 5 others. Of the 76 Coalition seats, 10 were Nationals, while there were 21 members of the Liberal National Party (ie in Queensland) elected.[91] The Nationals' policy is focused on 'regional Australia', which includes 'supporting Australia's farmers...'.[92] Clearly, then, without the support of the 'farmers' party', the Coalition would never gain government; the corollary is that the farmers of

---

[89] Watson (2014).
[90] Watson (2014).
[91] Australian Election Commission 2016 Federal Election. results.aec.gov.au/20499/Website/HouseDefault-20499.htm.
[92] National Party *What we stand for*. www.nationals.org.au/about.what-we-stand-for

Australia can exert political power out of proportion to their numbers or their contribution.

While there are many diverse bodies representing animal use industries, it is apparent those bodies have a very powerful influence in forming policy relating to animal welfare.[93] Chen (2016), conducted surveys of farming industry representatives and from his findings felt that most of the farming bodies had 'regular and enduring relationships with policy makers and regulators, such as key public servants, enforcement personnel...and politicians'.[94] He notes that this in effect keeps policy making out of the public gaze, and indeed away from scrutiny by parliaments; policy concerning animal use has thereby been captured by the farming lobby.

A key victory for the farming lobby occurred in 2013. The Liberal - National Coalition won government, and soon after Barnaby Joyce (then leader of the Nationals) was appointed as Minister for Agriculture. Joyce almost immediately dismantled any involvement of the federal government with animal welfare matters. Prior to that point, the federal government had served as coordinator of efforts to provide consistency on important questions such as animal welfare standards. At the time of writing, in early 2018, the situation is still chaotic.

With this move, and the subsequent statement that animal welfare was from then on to be dealt with at the states level, without any Federal leadership, Joyce effectively signalled an end to progress in animal welfare in agriculture. The federal Australian Animal Welfare Strategy (AAWS), which at that point had been running for several years, was abandoned. Whilst I (and many others interested in animal welfare) regarded AAWS as window dressing, with the benefit of hindsight, it is unfortunate to see some of the good work that was done being peremptorily dismissed. The extent of that work is indicated by an analysis of the agenda items in the Primary Industries Ministerial

---

[93] Chen (2016).
[94] Chen (2016).

Committee[95] from its inception, which shows that animal welfare was one of the top three most frequent items considered. Indeed, in 2003, the Committee noted its '...well-established role on animal welfare issues relating to production animals'.[96] This is clearly now not the case.

The policy of the national Labor Party differs substantially from the farmer-dominated, anti-animal welfare view pushed by the current Federal Coalition government. The Labor Party National Platform says 'increasingly, investors and consumers alike demand...respect for animal welfare standards' and (under the heading 'Animal welfare') *'All animals should be treated humanely. Labor will work to achieve better animal welfare and consistent application and enforcement of animal protection statutes by harmonising relevant federal, state and territory laws and codes. Labor will establish an independent office of animal welfare...and oppose any 'Ag-gag' legislation'*.[97] At present, these are words which are yet to be translated into any meaningful action. My own view, supported by all the available evidence, points to the Labor Party being terrified of upsetting farmers. For example, the backlash from the farming lobby following the brief suspension of live export in 2011 clearly spooked the Labor Party. The shadow spokesperson for agriculture, Joel Fitzgibbon, has described that decision as 'wrong', and has expressed concern about the fact that dairy farmers have told him they will never trust the Labor Party again. States Agriculture Ministers Alannah MacTiernan (Western Australia) and Jaala Pulford (Victoria), both in Labor governments, have indicated by their actions they take animal welfare seriously.[98]   However, it will be interesting to see

---

[95] This was a committee of all the states and territories ministers responsible for primary industry, and chaired by the federal agriculture minister.

[96] Botterill (2007).

[97] Labor Party National Platform www.alp.org.au/national_platform.

[98] Actions include reviews of the animal welfare legislation, indications that live exporters will be investigated for animal cruelty, and that battery cages for egg laying hens are unacceptable.

whether the federal Labor Party makes animal welfare a manifesto issue at the next federal election.

One might expect, that like environmental and other such issues, animal welfare would be a natural concern by those leaning towards the left side of politics. In fact, this is not the case. It seems that those who have concern about issues which are traditionally of interest to the left are not that interested in animal welfare. Artist and animal welfare commentator Yvette Watt has expressed the view that those committed to animal issues can be regarded as 'orphans of the left'. [99]

### The political power of the farming lobby

Farming bodies, although they are not interested in initiating improvements to animal welfare, nevertheless recognise it is regarded by much of the public as an important issue. For example, it appears that several organisations which represent the interests of animal users are seeking to address the question of animal welfare in their members' practices.[100]

While there is little doubt that farming organisations and other groups representing animal use industries have seriously inflated influence in policy making, there is a sense expressed by some in those groups that this could be a fragile position. The live export industry, for example, has repeatedly referred to its need to maintain a 'social licence'. The pig industry is seemingly conscious that consumers could easily lose confidence in the industry's ability to maintain adequate welfare standards, with serious negative consequences for pork producers.[101]

In my view, an important obstacle to progress in farm animal welfare is the powerful position of the state and federal departments of agriculture. These, at the same time, primarily service the interests of farmers, and have become increasingly responsible for making and

---

[99] Watt (2017).
[100] Chen (2016).
[101] Chen (2016).

enforcing the law governing animal enterprises. The exceptions are the ACT and South Australia; in the case of the latter state, the Department of Environment and Natural Resources has responsibility for animal welfare legislation.

Jed Goodfellow (2015)[102] has looked at this position from the point of view of the 'regulatory capture' of agencies which have the dual job of promoting farming interests, while also acting as 'animal welfare police'. He notes that those with vested interest in promoting animal use (the 'agricultural policy community') are regarded as being archetypal closed networks, with shared approaches to policy and an emphasis on excluding any competing views. Goodfellow interviewed several key officers in agriculture departments around the country. The responses he obtained confirmed several points, including that the roles of the departments were seen as promoting animal use industries and supporting their growth. Officers acknowledged that this gave rise to a conflict of interest when it came to looking after animal welfare; some referred to attempts to deal with this conflict by having different parts of the department dealing with industry support and promotion, as opposed to animal welfare. However, the real problem is evidenced by one regulator openly stating that there were forces within the department which would actively seek to protect the animal use industry from any possible sanctions in relation to breaches of animal welfare laws.

Goodfellow's work shows that regulators in agriculture departments are necessarily strongly influenced by the views of the Minister of the time and that the Minister in turn usually listens closely to the view of animal use organisations. There was said to be significant pressure from the animal use industry not to impose regulations. Animal welfare activities were uniformly underfunded. While regulators felt they had

---

[102] Respected animal welfare lawyer and academic who currently is RSPCA Australia's Policy Officer, but who has also worked in Queensland as an RSPCA inspector.

good working relationships with the animal use industry, their descriptions of animal protection groups was less positive, describing them as 'activists', 'extreme' and in one case, 'ferals'. It was the general view that animal protection groups did not understand the issues. There was strong evidence of a view that 'activists' were 'city-based' and so 'ignorant', whereas farmers had an accurate understanding of production and welfare issues. The 'city-country divide' is obviously alive and well. A rather shocking finding was that almost all of the regulators interviewed were unable to provide a coherent definition of 'animal welfare'. Several described 'animal welfare' as an 'emotional subject'. However, they had no difficulty expressing the idea that the real issue with animal welfare in the animal use industries was that good welfare should be targeted on increased productivity. Having said that, they understood that good productivity does not necessarily mean good welfare. None of the regulators made any reference to ethical considerations.

In conclusion, I believe that it is highly unlikely that there will be any significant improvements in the welfare of farmed animals until at least one major political party makes animal welfare an election issue. There is little evidence this is going to happen in the near future.

### Public concern about animal welfare in Australia

Who cares about animal welfare today? While it could be said that most Australians do care, animal welfare issues are not really a top priority, despite the large majority of Australians believing that animals are capable of thinking and feeling emotions.[103] Remarkably, Adrian Franklin (2007a) reported that a majority of Australians agreed with the proposition that animals should have the same moral rights as human beings. An unexpected source supporting the general thesis that there is significant public concern about animal welfare is the 2017

---

[103] Faunalytics Animal Tracker Australia – Baseline Report 2014.

Productivity Commission report,[104] *Regulation of Australian Agriculture*, which said

> '*animal welfare issues have received increased attention in Australia in recent years...the temporary suspension of live exports to Indonesia in 2011 is a prominent example...intensive farming and housing systems, such as stalls for pigs and cages for hens, have also been the subject of animal welfare campaigns. Exposure of incidents of mistreatment has raised community awareness and influenced consumers' attitudes*'.

This report rightly says that the community attaches a value to farm animal welfare that is distinct from the value that animal welfare contributes to the productivity and profitability of the farm business. This is a crucial distinction.

According to Jed Goodfellow (2015) the main proponents (from opposite sides of the philosophical fence) are what he calls the 'animal protection community', and the 'livestock industries'. These are the two groups which he rightly says are 'economically, morally or intellectually affected by government actions on farm animal welfare'.

I have little doubt that the attitude of the general public and the lawmakers who represent them has little or no tolerance of arguments that animals have rights of any kind, or that animal use and exploitation should cease. This necessarily colours the approach of animal advocacy organisations. While the RSPCAs have always stood by the idea that animals can be used providing they are humanely treated (the 'welfarist' view), organisations such as Animals Australia have never been wedded to that as a fundamental position. That said, Animals Australia's approach in recent years has been much more incrementalist in nature, pushing for things like humane slaughter, and

---

[104] The Productivity Commission is a federal government entity which provides independent research and advice to government on economic, social and environmental issues.

improvement of the conditions in which farmed animals are kept. It is clear that the only way organisations like Animals Australia will ever get traction with the public is to adopt a pragmatic strategy based on gradual improvement to animal welfare, with the tacit assumption that acceptance of use of animals must (at least for the time being) must be part of the strategy. Some academic commentators have adopted a critical tone of what may appear to them as acceptance by some key animal welfare figures such as Lyn White of Animals Australia of a 'welfarist' approach. This is, in my view, naive. For example Lyn White and Animals Australia could not adopt a strictly 'rightist' approach to the cruelty they reported in the Indonesian abattoirs shown in the *Four Corners* programme in 2011. If they had, there would have been far less impact, because most people accept slaughter of animals for food, but expect it to be done humanely. It is apparent that the public are disgusted by revelations of cruelty.

In recent times, the revelations of animal cruelty have often resulted from illegally obtained footage being given wide media attention. There have been many instances of such revelations in intensive pig and chicken facilities, as well as in sheep shearing sheds and abattoirs.[105] Brutal treatment of exported Australian sheep and cattle continues to be revealed. When these events are reported in the media, in every case members of the public express their outrage, farming groups inevitably refer to a few 'rogue operators' (or the like) giving the wrong impression, politicians make concerned noises, and then it is business as usual. In other words, the issue of animal welfare is one where there is public concern, but this does not translate to a meaningful political response.

Jed Goodfellow (2015) has prepared a useful commentary on the public attitudes to activists who carry out 'raids' (trespass) on facilities like intensive pig and poultry farms in order to gather evidence of cruelty. He points out that many of those involved in such activities, such as Lyn

---

[105] See references in Goodfellow (2015).

White of Animals Australia, and Mark Pearson (formerly of Animal Liberation), are highly regarded by the community, as evidenced by Lyn White receiving widespread praise for her revelations of cruelty in the live export industry, as well as being appointed a Member of the Order of Australia, and Mark Pearson's election to the Upper House of the New South Wales Parliament. The latter is a groundbreaking achievement for the first political party in Australia representing the interests of animals, the Animal Justice Party, to gain a parliamentary seat. But as Goodfellow points out, the other side of the coin is that many people (and not just those who have commercial interests in farming animals) disapprove of these 'direct actions'.

To summarise, I believe that in this country, we care about animals, but do not go so far in that caring to influence the politicians to do something, and counter the huge influence of the farming and animal use lobby. This is because, in the larger scheme, people are more concerned about other things, such as their childrens' education, health care and their general economic position, than animal welfare. There will not be real progress until animal welfare is regarded by the public as a really serious issue and politicians see it as something which will get them elected.

# Chapter 4   Animal welfare science

Properly conducted science can provide a valuable objective viewpoint on animal welfare issues. However, given the vested interests in animal use industries, it is a disturbing fact that in Australia much animal welfare science is paid for and controlled by the farming industry, or by the government departments whose main function is to look after those interests. The potential for conflict is self-evident.

Direct decisions in relation to animal welfare are taken by politicians, although consumers have an increasingly important role to play, as their viewpoints can influence what retailers are prepared to sell (see Chapter 11). In making their decisions, politicians (and to some extent retailers of animal products) can be informed by relevant science. But ultimately progress must be based on ethical and moral considerations.[106]

In this section I do not attempt to provide a definitive review of animal welfare science. However, I think even a superficial understanding of animal welfare science is very important for two main reasons. Firstly, knowledge of the science is essential in order to inform judgments about animal welfare legislation and policy, and secondly there has, in my view, been serious distortions in the Australian approach to animal welfare science for several decades now. I therefore present a focused and brief review of key scientific concepts and then demonstrate the flawed process of animal welfare science currently undertaken in Australia.

## History

'Animal welfare' is a term which has come into use only recently. According to Woods (2011), just 50 years ago, it rarely featured in public or political discourse. Things changed dramatically with the publication of Ruth Harrison's book *Animal Machines* in 1964. Although its author was not a scientist or veterinarian, it was 'thoroughly researched,

---

[106] Senate Animal Welfare Committee (1990).

closely argued and dispassionate in tone'.[107] It prompted a public outcry in the UK about intensive animal farming practices, particularly those relating to chickens, pigs and veal calves. Following intensive lobbying by the Royal Society for the Prevention of Cruelty to Animals, the response of the UK government was to appoint a committee under Professor FW Rogers Brambell FRS to investigate.[108] Importantly, the report had a separate annexe from one its members, WH Thorpe, who was an ethologist at Cambridge University.[109] This reflected the Committee's acceptance of the view that an animal's feelings were important.

Brambell explicitly identified the importance of using an anthropomorphic approach in a sensible fashion, acknowledging the undoubted similarities in anatomy and physiology which lead to the conclusion that many animals 'experience the same kinds of sensations as we do'. Critically, the Brambell Report drew parallels between human suffering and animal suffering. It accepted also that animals experience emotions, which include pleasure. It expressed concern about confinement for long periods which frustrated the ability of an animal to express its natural behaviour.

The ground-breaking report of that committee prompted the first animal welfare (as opposed to animal cruelty) legislation, followed by the introduction of codes of practice for those keeping livestock. This represented the first real use of the word 'welfare' in connection with animals, as distinct from the previous emphasis on 'cruelty' to animals.

The Farm Animal Welfare Advisory Committee was set up as a direct result of the Brambell Report. Its successor, the Farm Animal Welfare Council in 1979 set out the now well known 'Five Freedoms' (qualified

---

[107] Woods (2011).
[108] Woods (2011).
[109] Ethology is the science of animal behaviour.

by 'Five Provisions'), which reflected the principles identified in the Brambell Report. They are that an animal should have:

- Freedom from hunger and thirst, by ready access to fresh water and a diet to maintain full health and vigour.
- Freedom from discomfort, by providing an appropriate environment including shelter and a comfortable resting area.
- Freedom from pain, injury or disease, by prevention or rapid diagnosis and treatment.
- Freedom to express normal behaviour, by providing sufficient space, proper facilities and company of the animal's own kind.
- Freedom from fear and distress, by ensuring conditions and treatment which avoid mental suffering.[110]

It is interesting to note Woods' comment on the impact of Harrison's book, which still resonates today. The farmers' and the government's standard defence in these circumstances was to say that farmers were bound to look after their animals properly, as animals which suffered would be unable to grow and produce. Woods (2011) points out that farmers were operating on the assumption that they had something akin to an 'ancient contract' with animals. They looked after the animals, which in return provided product and profit. Harrison demonstrated that this was no longer so. The animal use industry today often goes quite close to acknowledging this constraint, referring to the need to have a 'social licence'. In other words, in the modern world, they cannot assume passive acceptance of whatever they choose to do.

Again resonating with things happening today, Harrison's opponents (ie the farmers) said that the science needed to look no further than productivity, and any other concern was 'subjective', 'emotional',

---

110

www.webarchive.nationalarchives.gov.uk/20121007104210/http:/www.fawc .org.uk.freedoms.htm. The 'Five Freedoms' were devised by Professor John Webster in 1979, when he joined the Farm Animal Advisory Committee, the precursor of FAWC: see Webster (2005) for a description of their genesis.

'anthropomorphic' and 'irrational'.[111] Despite this, the Brambell Report acknowledged the need to take into account the feelings of animals and expressly said it was permissible in this regard to refer to analogies based on human experience. It said to argue 'in the absence of any scientific method of evaluating whether an animal is suffering, its continued productivity should be taken as decisive evidence that it is not...is an over-simplified and incomplete view and we reject it'. Going further, the Report said 'it is morally incumbent upon us to give the animal the benefit of the doubt and to protect it so far as is possible from conditions that may be reasonably supposed to cause it suffering, though this cannot be proved'.

The UK government response to Brambell is analagous to the response of Australian governments today. It sought to dodge the recommendations and protect the interests of farmers. But influential members of Parliament resisted this, saying, for example 'we will never have legislation to protect animals if we must know first how much pain they have in all circumstances'.[112]

Prominent animal welfare scientist Professor Donald Broom has provided a useful review of the development of animal welfare science post-Brambell. As part of that, he emphasises the importance of identifying the needs of animals, and refers to studies in the 1970s and 1980s of livestock in 'natural' environments which showed that many farm animal breeds were, in behavioural terms, 'scarcely distinguishable in many respects from that of their wild ancestors'.[113]

## What is animal welfare science?
Before talking about animal welfare science, it is necessary to ask what 'animal welfare' is. Broom (1986) defined animal welfare, saying it is the animal's state 'as regards its attempt to cope with its environment.' This is a useful scientific definition, because it regards animal welfare as a

---

[111] Woods (2011).
[112] Woods (2011).
[113] Broom (2011).

measurable parameter, which can range on a scale from bad to good. However, it has been criticised on the grounds that it does not define what relevant stimuli influencing welfare might be, nor does it say what is good or bad welfare.[114] Marian Dawkins has advanced a simpler definition, which she feels is readily understood by non-scientists, as well as aligning with other animal welfare system definitions, such as Welfare Quality. She says that good welfare is when an animal is healthy and has what it wants.[115] John Webster also notes that an important question is whether an animal is happy and healthy, and additionally asks whether the animal is living a natural life – the latter qualified by establishing whether the animal is in an environment consistent with one in which the species evolved and to which it has adapted.[116]

An animal which is unable to cope may suffer serious consequences, such as a failure to grow, reproduce or indeed continue living. These consequences are at the extreme end of the spectrum. An animal may suffer none of these, but still spend a significant amount of time in extreme suffering and thereby be in a state of very poor welfare.

There are many measures which animal welfare scientists can make which may give indications of the state of welfare of an animal. The main measures are of physiological changes, behaviour, health status, injury, growth and reproduction and life expectancy. These have recently been put together as a conceptual framework under the headings of 'biological functioning', 'affective state' and 'natural living'.[117] The emphasis until quite recently, particularly in Australia (and driven by the influential group at the University of Melbourne), has been on measures related to 'biological functioning', with de-emphasis of measures designed to assess subjective experiences or affects.

---

[114] Webster (2005).
[115] Dawkins (2017b).
[116] Webster (2005).
[117] see Hemsworth et al. (2015); Mellor (2016b)..

As I have already noted (and it is worth repeating), the Brambell Report as long ago as 1965 was dismissive of the idea that an animal showing good productivity was in a good state of welfare. It referred to submissions which maintained that any suffering would be reflected in a corresponding fall in productivity; continued productivity should be taken as decisive evidence that an animal is not suffering. The Committee's response to this was to say 'this is an over-simplified and incomplete view and we reject it'.

This 'over-simplified' view still prevails in some quarters.[118] This is to be expected, as a person running a business where an animal is the saleable commodity (directly or indirectly) will want to maintain that commodity in a state where financial returns are maximised. This position is not one shared by the international consensus of animal welfare scientists, which is that an animal can be very productive, and husbandry can be good, but the animal can be in a state of poor welfare.[119]

One of the fundamental difficulties facing animal welfare scientists is how much weight to give each measure indicating the state of welfare of an animal. As the Brambell Report pointed out, this is a matter of balanced judgment. It took the view that factors producing prolonged animal welfare problems may be of much more significance than more acute, albeit transitory suffering. But this really does not address the thorny problem. As an illustration, it will be seen that egg-laying chickens kept in free-range systems may experience higher rates of mortality than birds kept in battery cages (although there is some debate about this). However, it goes without saying that the birds kept in free range systems are better able to express natural behaviours. So what weight should be given to each parameter? Is it better to give an animal more freedom to move about, interact with other animals, and

---

[118] see the survey data in Chen (2016). See also Esther Han 'Egg industry rebuked for claiming that unhappy hens won't produce eggs' *Sydney Morning Herald* 7 March 2017.
[119] see for example Webster (2005).

express natural behaviours, while possibly shortening its life span? Questions like these are rarely addressed – or in the case of some scientists, the 'physiological' measures, particularly of so-called stress hormones, are given substantial and inappropriate weight.

It is important not to forget the qualification that sometimes science might get ahead of itself. Weary et al. (2016) give the example of the modified (or furnished) cage for layer hens. As they say, this is 'an elegant scientific solution', which unfortunately did not fulfil the requirements of many of those concerned about animal welfare, not least of which is the general public. While European legislation has imposed a requirement for furnished cages, it is safe to say that this has not resonated with the general public, which is far likelier to prefer the idea of hens being kept 'free range', and to regard a cage, whether furnished or not, as still being a cage, and thereby unacceptable.

## Stress

The concept of stress is regarded by some as particularly important in animal welfare science. A measure of stress has been a major driver of research. There is a fairly widely held view among scientists that stress may be measured by assay of the output of 'stress hormones', which are glucocorticoid steroids. Cortisol is one such hormone (in chickens the relevant hormone is a related molecule, corticosterone). It is produced by the adrenal cortex, in response to intermediate hormones from the pituitary gland (located at the base of the brain), which in turn receives stimulatory signals from the brain region known as the hypothalamus. This is referred to as the hypothalamic-pituitary-adrenal cortex, or HPA system. Cortisol has effects on various target tissues with the overall result of providing extra energy for forthcoming activity in response to a stimulus, which may include a stressful stimulus. For example, cortisol levels increase in response to feeding, hardly a stressful situation.[120]

---

[120] Mormede et al. (2007).

Many take the view that an increase in 'stress' is an indicator of poor welfare. Broom and Johnson (2007) rightly point out that this view is simplistic and misleading. Increases in HPA activity in animals can be seen in many situations which would not be regarded as associated with poor welfare, including courtship, mating and catching prey. Webster (2005) remarks that when he put his dog (and his children) in the car to go to the seaside, they all got excited. He rightly surmises that the excitement will be associated with an increase in cortisol. The same would be observed with farm animals loaded onto a vehicle. So how does one distinguish the 'good' cortisol (going to the seaside and excited at the prospect) from the 'bad' cortisol (possibly having a bad experience being transported on a truck)? The answer, of course, is you can't.

## Needs

Animals have needs and if those needs are unsatisfied an animal's welfare will be compromised.[121] Examples include the need to have an adequate state of nutrition, a comfortable temperature and social interactions. These needs are controlled by various functional systems. Body temperature, for instance, is tightly controlled in homoeothermic animals (such as mammals or birds) by specific physiological mechanisms. So a need is a requirement (part of the basic biology of the animal) to obtain a particular resource (such as food or water) or respond to a particular environmental or bodily stimulus (for example responding to heat by activating physiological mechanisms to keep cool, such as sweating, or engaging in a behaviour such as seeking shade).

Examples of needs in farm animals are the need for pigs to root in soil (or similar), or hens' need to dustbathe; both these species also need to build nests before giving birth or laying eggs. Denying the animals these needs probably results in poor welfare.[122]

---

[121] see Dawkins (2017a).
[122] Broom and Fraser (2007).

Needs can be identified by careful study of animals in a 'natural' environment.[123] That is not to say that 'being natural' is necessary for good animal welfare. It is not.[124] Natural behaviour may point to possible welfare issues, but it is not on its own a reliable indicator.[125] Indeed, animals in a natural environment may suffer considerably.[126] More recently, careful use of choice experiments have allowed researchers to make useful conclusions about animals' preferences. This gives insight into 'what animals want'.[127]

## Sentience

The question of sentience in animals is gaining increasing attention. This is an important question because it relates back directly to the questions of animal suffering and contentment. Animal suffering and contentment can only assume importance if the animal concerned is able to appreciate that it is suffering, or is happy or otherwise. This is the issue which was implicit in Bentham's question as to whether an animal could suffer.[128] Webster, taking these words as a guide, suggests one can say a sentient animal is one 'for whom feelings matter'.[129] This at least focuses one on the meaning of the feelings to the animal. But it still does not say where the bar should be set.

The greater importance from the point of view of a law-maker is that if one accepts the need to minimise suffering and maximise contentment for animals, then the threshold question requires definition of which animals can appreciate their state. This remains an important scientific issue and there is a great degree of variation in the attribution of emotions to animals. The 'functional category' of an animal is

---

[123] eg chickens: McBride et al. (1969); pigs: Wood-Gush et al. (1990).

[124] Broom (2011).

[125] Dawkins (2017a).

[126] Webster (2005) gives the example of high piglet mortality in 'natural' situations. As he says, referring to this as just a production problem 'rather devalues the distress associated with dying'.

[127] Dawkins (2017a).

[128] Chapter 3.

[129] Webster (2005).

influential, as is an animal's perceived place in the hierarchy of species. This highlights the need to translate the scientific views on sentience to wider public awareness.[130]

Animals have different levels of self-awareness, and their awareness of their interactions with their environment. This different level of ability includes the ability to experience pleasurable states, as well as aversive states. 'Sentience', in this context, usually means the animal concerned has the awareness and cognitive ability enabling it to have feelings. This raises the question as to which abilities an animal must have in order to be 'sentient'. Professor Donald Broom has said *'a sentient being is one that has some ability: to evaluate the actions of others in relation to itself and third parties, to remember some of its own actions and their consequences, to assess risk, to have some feelings and to have some degree of awareness.'*[131]

Sentience is not consciousness. Consciousness refers to a wide range of states in which there is an immediate awareness of thought, image or sensation. The basic experiences of sensation (seeing, hearing, feeling pain, etc) are what has been described as phenomenal consciousness and sentience is the ability to have these experiences.[132] Note that even defining the neuronal basis of 'consciousness' is currently regarded as very difficult if not impossible;[133] as Dawkins (2017a) says: '...we will have a healthier biological approach to the study of consciousness if we acknowledge the uncomfortable, inconvenient and unsatisfactory truth that conscious awareness is still an unsolved problem'. The issue of consciousness in animals becomes even more problematic when one considers the potential multiplicity of systems which could underlie 'consciousness', let alone the pitfalls of extrapolating from one species to another.[134] One of the major difficulties is for humans to understand

---

[130] Wilkins et al. (2015).
[131] See Broom and Fraser (2007).
[132] Dawkins (2006).
[133] Baars and Edelman (2012).
[134] Dawkins (2017a).

the conscious state or feelings of animals. In the absence of language (ie, with animals) that is a particular problem.[135] Many people are prepared to attribute higher mental abilities to mammalian species, but feel reluctant to do so with many other species. Birds, for example, are typically regarded as not having many mental skills. However, there is good evidence from a variety of disciplines to support the view that non-mammalian species, including several bird species have higher order consciousness.[136] Despite their brain structure being very different from that of mammals, cephalopods such as the octopus and cuttlefish have sophisticated cognitive abilities.[137] The need to analyse sentience is illustrated by the position regarding fish. It is apparent that most members of the public are indifferent to fish welfare; salmon, for example, were rated as having limited mental abilities, including the ability to feel pain.[138] Contrast this with the scientific analysis: Broom and Fraser (2007) conclude that fish have abilities indicating they are sentient, including awareness of what is happening around them, cognitive processing capacity and the ability to feel pain. Some fish species have mental representations of their environment (necessary in relation to navigation abilities) and can learn spatial relationships. Fish have complex learning abilities and can probably feel fear.[139] The argument that fish lack the mammalian neural mechanisms responsible for the pain sensation uses flawed anthrophomorphic analysis. That is not the question; the important issue is whether one puts together all the evidence, it points in the direction that fish can feel pain.[140]

Broom (2014) makes the point that it is common for people to assume that animals are somehow inferior to humans on the grounds that humans have unique qualities. These may include having a 'soul', or some such, and possessing 'free will'. Another idea is that humans have

---

[135] Edelman and Seth (2009).
[136] Edelman and Seth (2009).
[137] Edelman and Seth (2009).
[138] Kupsala et al. (2013).
[139] See also Broom (2007).
[140] see Burghardt (2016).

a 'mind', which in the past, as with the 'soul', might be regarded as somehow separate from the physical body. That is not a sustainable concept. Mind is a function of the brain, and the existence of a 'soul' is a matter of opinion.

A further bias is that of humans assuming that animals which are similar to humans in form and function are likely to be sentient. Consequently, fish, reptiles, insects, spiders and molluscs receive little respect in this context.[141]

It is of central importance, therefore, to know which characteristics an animal should possess in order to be regarded as sentient. It follows that animals which are sentient are those whose welfare needs to be protected. The task of animal welfare science is to assess whether animals possess awareness, are capable of cognitive processing, and can have feelings, such as pain. Other evidence which can be considered includes complexity of life and behaviour, learning ability, functioning of brain and nervous system, and identification of a biological basis of suffering and other feelings such as fear and anxiety.[142]

So the question remains as to where to set the bar. Kirkwood (2006) refers to the incorporation into European Union legislation of the wording that there should be provision '...to ensure improved protection and respect for the welfare of animals as sentient beings'. This is wide of the mark, because all animals are not sentient. A better wording would refer to 'the welfare of sentient animals'. Animal species represent about 5% of all living species. They have the characteristics of being multicellular, and eating other life forms. This leaves open the issue of which animals are sentient and which are not. Many simple organisms respond by moving towards food, or moving away from threats, with sensory systems that give them relevant information, and with processing systems enabling them to remember these sorts of things. But that does not mean they are sentient. Kirkwood (2006)

---

[141] Broom (2014).
[142] Broom and Littin, cited in Broom (2007).

argues that, because the determination of whether an animal is sentient or not is morally important, we should give all animals the benefit of the doubt and treat them as if they are sentient. I fear this is going too far.

As Broom (2014) has said, there is a general view that there is a threshold level among animals above which an animal is deserving of protection by the law. It is easy to say that protozoans or nematode worms (for example) are below the threshold, and that primates are above the level, but what about those in between? Broom's view is that there is a continually changing and advancing state of knowledge regarding the abilities and level of functioning of non-human animals, so there must be an ongoing reappraisal of where that line should be drawn. Arguably, animals less able to cope with pain (for example) because they have a less complex brain may suffer worse welfare for a given 'level' of pain than an animal which is better equipped (by virtue of its more complex processing ability) to cope.

Another outstanding issue is the ontogeny of sentience. Many painful procedures, such as castration or de-horning of cattle, which have been routinely carried out without pain relief, have been justified on the basis that they can be done on very young animals because they are less sentient than older animals. The true justification may be that the younger animals are easier to restrain, heal quicker and may be less likely to remember the procedure. But obviously the real question is how sentient are they?[143]

I am inclined to the view put by Marian Dawkins, that sentience is the 'hard problem' because we do not know what it is, where it comes from, what it does or where to find it in other species.[144] Because of that, it may be a dangerous distraction when making decisions about which species of animals require protection. Perhaps the safe view, worth repeating, is to err on the side of caution.

---

[143] Duncan (2006).
[144] Dawkins (2006).

But regardless of where we set the bar for sentience, I agree with Karen Davis (2017) that there is a big risk in ranking animals in this way. In particular, the effort to persuade courts to grant great apes 'personhood' in the Nonhuman Rights Project, led by Steven Wise, is, I think, misguided. Success could have a seriously negative effect, being the reinforcement of the attitudes and speciesism which have entrenched the miserable position of so many animals.

## Statistics

Statistical analysis is crucial for the objective interpretation of scientific data. Objectivity is particularly important in animal welfare science where so often the results of a study can determine whether or not many hundreds of thousands of animals continue to spend their lives in poor conditions. The confinement of chickens to a life spent in battery cages, or of female pigs to a life spent in sow stalls and farrowing crates are two obvious examples. The animal use industry often relies on animal welfare science to justify practices which many would find cruel; that science is frequently paid for by the industry. It is therefore necessary to be especially critical in assessing whether animal welfare science data mean what the experimenters say they mean. In recent years there has been an upsurge of criticism of scientific research publications in general, exemplified by John Ioannidis' 2005 article *Why most published research findings are false*. This applies *a fortiori* to animal welfare science research.

The statistical approach adopted by almost all experimental scientists, and certainly all animal welfare scientists, is to firstly construct a 'null hypothesis'. An example of a null hypothesis would be 'stress hormone levels are the same regardless of whether chickens are kept in battery cages, or kept in a free range system'. Because biological measures are intrinsically variable from animal to animal, scientists have to make repeated measures in a sample group – this is simply because it is impossible to make measures in all the population of subject animals. That means scientists have to decide on how many samples to take. This is a very important consideration, because the greater the sample number, the more confidence you can have that any difference(s) you see between groups (in the example, free ranging versus caged chickens) are real. Because one is taking samples, it is necessary to have a measure of 'central tendency' in each group of samples. The most frequently used measure is the arithmetic mean, or average (most commonly referred to as 'the mean'). In the example given, it would be highly unlikely that the mean stress hormone levels in the two experimental groups (that is, battery cages versus free range) would be identical, because of intrinsic variability between individuals (to understand intrinsic variability, think of the range of heights of a random sample of people). That being so, the null hypothesis is that the true value of the difference between the means is zero. The scatter, or range, of the individual observations in the samples can be calculated, and is usually expressed as a parameter based on the difference of the observations from the mean value. One such commonly used parameter is the 'standard error of the mean' (often just called 'standard error').

In doing statistical analysis, a scientist will calculate a value for $P$. If the result is that the value of $P$ is 0.05, one can say:

> If there were actually no effect (if the true difference between means were zero) then the probability of observing a value for the difference equal to, or greater than, that actually observed would be $P = 0.05$. In other words there is a 5% chance of seeing a difference at least as big as we have done, by chance alone.[145]

David Colquhoun has pithily said 'at first sight, it might be thought that this procedure would guarantee that you would make a fool of yourself only once in every 20 times that you do a test. But it implies nothing of the sort...'.[146] This is because the classical $P$ value is a statement about what would happen if there were no true effect. In fact, sometimes there really is an effect. The first thing to know is the probability that

---

[145] Colquhoun (2014).
[146] Colquhoun (2014).

the test will give the right result when there is a real effect. This is called the 'power' of the test, which increases as the sample size increases. The sample size is often set so that a real effect is detected in 80% of tests. Colquhoun (2014) shows how, using these experimental analysis choices, one ends up with a false discovery rate of 36%, not 5%. As he says 'it is...clear that if you use $P=0.05$ as a magic cut off point, you are very likely to make a fool of yourself by claiming a real effect when there is none.' He suggests 'if you want to avoid making a fool of yourself very often, do not regard anything greater than $P<0.001$ (ie the 1% level) as a demonstration that you have discovered something.'

There is another major problem which is prevalent in the animal welfare science literature. This is where scientists carry out a statistical analysis, get a $P$ value a little greater than 0.05 (5%) and say the difference between means is 'almost significant', has a 'tendency to significant' or any other 'time-honoured tactic of circumlocution to disguise the non-significant result as something more interesting.'[147] This is deeply misleading, to quote Colquhoun (2014). It amounts to 'spinning' the results.[148] Unfortunately, the practice is commonplace in animal welfare science publications. This means that animal welfare science research must be scrutinised very carefully in order to assess the validity of conclusions made by authors.

Broom and Fraser (2007) make the powerful point that in studies of animal behaviour where one is looking at groups of animals, it is important to be able to identify individual animals. This is because treating animals as having a mean or average behaviour may completely miss behaviours which are quite different in a significant number of individuals.

### Measures of animal welfare

Estimating an animal's welfare status requires a view of the whole animal, and requires measurement of many parameters. While such

---

[147] Motulsky (2015).
[148] See Boutron et al. (2010).

measurement may include consideration of growth and reproductive success (ie what a farmer would call 'productivity'), that measure alone cannot be relied upon to indicate whether an animal's welfare is good or bad. It is beyond doubt that an animal can show good productivity, while still having poor welfare.

Poor welfare can be indicated by poor health (including injury and disease), growth or reproductive ability.[149] Dawkins (2017a) has rightly pointed out that many improvements in animal welfare have been achieved with a focus on health, without even the need to believe that animals are conscious or experience feelings.

The problem for those attempting to quantify animal welfare is the integration of whatever measures they make, tempered with the knowledge that measurement of merely physical elements (that is, physiology, behaviour, health, productivity, etc) may miss welfare problems which are purely mental. An obvious example is depression.[150]

*Physiology*

For many years, there has been a very strong tendency in scientific studies of animal welfare, particularly in influential Australian work, to emphasise the importance of 'physiological' measures.[151] Such measures might include measurement of heart rate, blood pressure, levels of particular blood cells, or of glucocorticoids (the so-called 'stress hormones').

The emphasis on measurement of glucocorticoids, which has dominated Australian animal welfare science for decades, while de-emphasising measures relating to behaviour, is exemplified by the statement in 1990 by Dr John Barnett to the Senate Animal Welfare inquiry into intensive farming, when he said

---

[149] Broom (1996).
[150] Marchant-Forde (2009a).
[151] Hagan et al. (2011)

*'...so physiologically when we assess stress in animals we say that there is evidence that these animals are stressed from hormone measurements. But that does not mean their welfare is at risk. You then go and look at the consequences to the animal of that change in hormone level. If you start finding consequences which can be indicative of nutritional problems or energy problems by going to energy deficit; it has effects on the immune system; it has effects on production. Once you start finding those effects of the consequence of stress you say, who is at risk? That is what we are trying to do physiologically. Behaviourally I do not think they are so advanced'.*

This statement is telling for two reasons. First, it implies that a change in glucocorticoids does not by itself indicate poor welfare. One has to go to other measures to draw that conclusion. This statement is entirely rational. However, the second reason for remarking on this passage is it would be fine were it not for the fact that the principle expressed was and is ignored in practice, not least by Dr Barnett and his colleagues. Small changes in glucocorticoid levels (quite frequently not even passing the usual accepted test for statistical significance) are routinely said to indicate poor welfare, or more disturbingly, no increases in these 'stress hormones' are erroneously interpreted as showing good welfare. This has been the subject of outspoken criticism by some (non-Australian) animal welfare scientists.[152]

While there is little doubt that serious derangement of any of these physiological parameters may be indicative of poor welfare, equally, an emphasis on such measurements when the question relates to the mental state of the animal is likely to be very misleading. It hardly needs saying that something as complex as feelings of frustration, anxiety, depression or wellbeing cannot be measured by looking at the level of some hormone. Nevertheless, there has been an explosion of studies using such measures, particularly those measuring glucocorticoids. My

---

[152] eg Rushen (1991).

own view is that this has been stimulated by two main factors, the first being that scientists can market these measures as being highly technical and thereby impressive (as opposed to merely observing an animal's behaviour, which sounds rather trivial and easy) and the second being that (in fact) they are technically relatively easy to make. John Webster has described them as 'dangerously easy'.[153]

Increased HPA activity as a result of stress can lead to increased levels of the glucocorticoids cortisol (in most mammals; corticosterone in birds). As noted, this can only be interpreted as signifying poor welfare if it is differentiated from rises in these hormones associated with generalized arousal. Rises in 'stress hormones' occur not only when there may be reduced welfare, but also in anticipation of food, sex, access to improved environments and other situations normally associated with positive emotions.[154] This is a fact which is routinely ignored. Absence of an increase in glucocorticoid level at a particular time after a treatment or action does not necessarily mean the animal is not suffering stress. This is because the classic pattern of glucocorticoid response to stress is a fairly rapid rise, followed by a gradual decline back to basal levels as the glucocorticoid stores in the adrenal gland become exhausted.[155] Moreover, there is strong evidence that cortisol levels not only have a circadian rhythm, but also change in a pulsatile fashion on a minute by minute basis, with the profile differing greatly between different animals. Where the stressor is present chronically, the cortisol levels are not maintained, but instead decline.[156] Taken together, this means that attempts to measure cortisol at a single time point, and use this as an indicator of an animal's welfare status, are likely to be meaningless.[157] Other measures, such as behavioural measures, may indicate that the animal is still experiencing poor welfare, even though glucocorticoid levels appear normal. This

---

[153] Webster (2005).
[154] See Dawkins (2017a); Spencer and Deak (2017).
[155] Mormede et al. (2011).
[156] Broom and Fraser (2007); Spencer and Deak (2017).
[157] Ladewig and Smidt (1989);

means that a change in 'stress hormones' is meaningless unless it is correlated with another measure (for example a behavioural indicator) which indicates the 'valence' of the response. In other words, something the animal wants: positive valence, or something it wants to get away from: negative valence. Dawkins (2017a) summarises it thus:

> *'the physiological changes in the animal's body tell us that it is responding to something but by themselves are often ambiguous, indicating merely that the animal is preparing for action of some sort but without telling us information whether it is preparing to run towards or away from something'.*

When glucocorticoid levels are measured in blood, the very act of taking a blood sample can cause stress to the animal which itself will increase glucocorticoid release.[158] This sampling artefact makes the use of non-invasive measures of glucocorticoid levels attractive. These have included using faeces, saliva or (for birds) eggs and feathers. Theoretically at least these procedures may offer the additional advantage that the relatively transient response of plasma glucocorticoid becomes integrated into the indirect measure. But in the absence of direct proof this is the case, this remains speculative. Furthermore, there are serious technical difficulties involved in these measures.

It has been said that increased glucocorticoid levels can lead to suppression of the immune system. This certainly happens for example where humans have been treated with high levels of artificial steroids, such as prednisone. But that is different from saying that any observed increase in glucocorticoid levels necessarily has a detrimental effect on an animal's health status. To claim that, a scientist must provide evidence – in this case, of impairment of immune function which means something to the animal. This does not amount to just measuring the ratio of certain white blood cells and saying it has changed. One must

---

[158] Wein et al. (2017).

consider whether or not a clinical assessment would conclude that the parameters are outside the normal ranges.

Webster (2005) quotes an excellent example from the work of McFarlane and colleagues which illustrates how taking any one of these physiological measures of indicating animal welfare status has the potential to be entirely misleading. In the studies he refers to, growing chicks were exposed to several stressors, either alone or in combination. The stressors included increased levels of ammonia, infection with the organism *Coccidia*, elevated temperature causing heat stress and electric shock. None of these stressors increased the level of stress hormone (corticosterone); the infection, which would be expected to stimulate the immune system, did not cause any change in the ratio of white blood cells normally regarded as indicating the status of the immune system. However, what the stressors, when combined, did change was weight gain, food intake and food conversion efficiency – all were reduced. This just shows how completely misleading physiological measures can be when taken In isolation.

Recently, some influential animal welfare scientists have said that it is the biological cost of stress that is the key to understanding the associated welfare implications.[159] The extent of an animal's coping with challenges is reflected in the normality of its biological functioning, they say. Personally, I think this is easy to say, and much harder to put into practice in a way which is really meaningful.

### Behaviour

Today's leading animal welfare scientists regard measures of behaviour as critical to the understanding of an animal's welfare status.[160] That was not always the case.

It took a considerable time before study of animal behaviour was even recognised as being important and relevant in assessing animal welfare.

---

[159] Hemsworth et al. (2015).
[160] See Webster (2005).

The domination of experimental psychology by the 'behaviorist' thoughts and techniques of JB Watson and Skinner set animal behaviour studies back many years.[161] Underlying this was the notion that animal consciousness was beyond scientific examination. Watson famously said:

> 'psychology as the behaviorist views it is a purely objective experimental branch of natural science. Its theoretical goal is the prediction and control of behavior. Introspection forms no essential part of its methods, nor is the scientific value of its data dependent upon the readiness with which they lend themselves to interpretation in terms of consciousness.'

The kernel of this argument was that 'feelings' were irrelevant. One can see Cartesian echoes of 'animal as machine' here. Skinner's opinion was 'we seem to have an inside information about our behavior – we have feelings about it. And what a diversion they have proved to be...feelings have proved to be one of the most fascinating attractions along the path of dalliance'.[162] The Skinnerian school of thought has been rejected by most psychologists over the last few decades,[163] although anti-anthropomorphism is still axiomatic.[164] But powerful arguments have been made for the application of 'critical anthropomorphism' to the study of animal behaviour, which seems entirely logical.[165]

One cannot make deductions about what animals feel while pretending not to impose one's own views and experiences. The attribution of mental states is partially founded on common mental and behavioural substrates in humans and other animals.[166] The braver animal welfare scientists point out that where one is talking about assessing these sort

---

[161] see Duncan (2006).
[162] Duncan, chapter 5, in Benson and Rollin (2004).
[163] Duncan (2006).
[164] Kennedy (1992).
[165] Burghardt (2007).
[166] Urquiza-Haas et al. (2015).

of things, there is no objective human observer, as scientists are part of the overall reality and hence there is no position which is 'perspective free'. In other words, one cannot avoid some colouration by anthropomorphism.[167]

In any case, the assessment of an animal's feelings is, by definition, impossible. All one can attain is an estimate, an indication. This does not mean that the attempt to assess feelings is futile; rather it means one must be very careful. John Webster (2005) summarises it nicely: *'You would think me presumptuous if I were to speak with authority on how you feel. Thus we may both conclude that any attempt by us to define how a cow or a rat may feel is a matter to be approached with extreme caution.'*

The assessment of animal behaviour requires knowledge of many things, including how an animal senses what is going on in its environment. Animals may be very different from humans in this regard – the most obvious difference is the much greater importance of olfaction (smell) to animals than to humans. There are other important differences which must be taken into account, such as the ability of some animals to hear different frequencies of sound, or light (Broom and Fraser, 2007).

There is an important question regarding an animal's 'feelings'. Some workers have emphasised the importance of feelings in determining whether an animal's welfare is good or bad;[168] others have said feelings are important, but not exclusively so. John Webster (2005) puts it thus: 'the welfare of any sentient animal is determined by its individual perception of its own physical and emotional state'. I find it hard to disagree with this. Professor Donald Broom's definition of welfare has been attacked as not sufficiently emphasising the role of an animal's feelings; however, he is of the view that his definition of welfare encompasses the need to consider feelings. That seems entirely

---

[167] Wemelsfelder et al. (2000).
[168] see Duncan and Petherick (1991).

reasonable.[169] While pain, fear and other negative feelings have been regarded for a long time as important in animal welfare assessment, it is only more recently that the incidence (or the encouragement or promotion of) positive feelings has been recognised as important.[170] Marian Dawkins (2017a) thinks that one should not get overly focused on animal feelings; she feels that it is possible to make important deductions about animal welfare, based, for example on choice experiments (to identify needs), or measures of what keeps animals healthy, which make no assumptions about feelings or even consciousness in the animal.[171]

It is also important to remember that an animal in a poor state of health is probably also not feeling good. For example, a severe infection is associated with release of powerful inflammatory mediators (as the immune system responds to fight the infection). This is what makes a person feel ill when they are infected and there is every reason to believe an animal will undergo the same experience.[172]

Poor welfare can be inferred when an animal strongly avoids an object or situation, and *vice versa*. The presence of abnormal behaviours such as stereotypies, self-mutilation, tail-biting in pigs and feather pecking in hens are indicative of poor welfare. Stereotypies are of particular interest, as they are often manifest where animals are closely confined. A stereotypy is a repeated, relatively invariant sequence of movements that has no obvious function.[173] Sows confined in sow stalls will often spend several hours carrying out such behaviour: an example is repeated pushing of a drinker nipple, without actually drinking. Another example in caged pregnant sows is bar-biting. It seems that these

---

[169] See Broom (2011).
[170] Broom (2014).
[171] Dawkins (2017a). See also Dawkins (1990).
[172] Webster (2005).
[173] Broom and Fraser (2007).

behaviours in pigs can be reduced if the animal is given increased food rations, or manipulable material (eg straw).[174]

Another form of abnormal behaviour seen in farmed pigs is tail-biting. This can result in serious damage to a pig due to contamination of the wounds, with spread of infection to other parts of the body. The conditions that predispose animals to biting the tails of other animals include dense grouping of pigs during their rapid growth phase, insufficient trough space and drinking facilities and adverse environmental factors (eg high noise levels).[175] Intensive pig farmers have developed the practice of tail docking, conducted on young piglets without pain relief, to reduce tail biting.

Pain is an important consideration in assessing animal welfare. Pain is useful to an animal as it alerts the animal to potential harm and allows the animal to escape from harmful stimuli.[176] However, it is axiomatic that if an animal is suffering chronic and serious pain, its welfare is poor. It is also obvious (as any veterinarian will tell you) that one can only say an animal is in pain on the basis of indirect measures: an animal cannot tell you it is in pain. Behavioural changes indicative of pain are therefore indispensable in animal welfare assessment. Broom and Fraser (2007) give several examples of such behaviours. One such is vocalization. This happens with social animals such as pigs and dogs, probably because it is part of the communication within a social group, where group members may help individuals in pain. But this is not so with prey species, possibly because vocalizations may attract predators. Another example of a response to chronic and severe pain is evidence of altered mood. Webster (2005) gives the example of the meat chicken suffering from locomotor disorders which show a decrease in grooming activities and eating. He also references work from the Bristol animal welfare science group showing that chickens exhibiting symptoms of lameness

---

[174] Broom and Fraser (2007).
[175] Broom and Fraser (2007).
[176] Webster (2005).

will elect to eat food containing an analgesic drug, while those not so suffering will choose the undrugged food. All of this is convincing evidence of the extent to which the pain matters to these animals. It is worth noting that animal welfare scientists have devised pain scales to allow the estimation of the extent of pain a particular member of an animal species is suffering. One of the best known of these is the Glasgow scale, developed for dogs.

Preventing a behaviour which an animal is motivated to carry out will also possibly result in reduced welfare. This is illustrated by the desire of chickens to flap their wings at intervals, which they cannot do in battery cages. Likewise, sows kept in stalls or farrowing crates on concrete or slatted floors are prevented from engaging in rooting or nest-building behaviour.[177]

Observations of what an animal chooses to do, when faced with choices, may be a useful way of deciding what to provide for an animal in its environment. For example, hens prefer to stand on a floor which gives greatest support to their toes, rather than on a rigid floor.[178]

As well as identifying ways to avoid causing problems for animals, it is also important to recognise that changes can be made to maximise positive feelings in animals, and this effect is susceptible to measurement.[179] It may even be that behaviour which has previously been regarded as need-driven (such as dust-bathing in chickens) is in fact pleasurable.[180]

## Species-related welfare issues

### Pigs
Held et al. (2009) reviewed knowledge of cognition and emotion in pigs and concluded that there were sensory faculties, cognitive abilities and

---

[177] Broom and Fraser (2007).
[178] Broom and Fraser (2007).
[179] Broom (2011).
[180] Duncan (2006).

behavioural priorities in domestic pigs that would have helped their wild ancestors survive and reproduce optimally under natural conditions. Importantly, these authors felt that pigs kept today for pork production seem to have retained many of these faculties, and may therefore be behaviourally, cognitively and emotionally at odds with the intensively husbanded environment they spend their lives in.

The modern pig breeds used for pork production grow very rapidly, and this has led to increased bone problems, such as decreased bone strength and leg weakness.[181] It also appears that selection of pigs for rapid muscle growth has resulted in an increase in the incidence of tail biting.[182] Pregnant sows are often fed concentrated diets, requiring their feed intake to be restricted in order to prevent obesity. In all likelihood, these animals are in a chronic state of hunger, which promotes aberrant behaviours such as bar-biting.[183]

It goes without saying that carrying out mutilations such as teeth clipping and tail docking on piglets would be expected to cause pain. The scientific evidence supports this view.[184] Early weaning of piglets has been said to potentially lead to digestive disorders and predisposition to infection.[185]

There have been detailed studies of the behaviour of pigs in 'natural' environments, which is helpful in terms of defining the 'needs' of pigs.[186]

Sows housed in stalls experience physical and mental health problems. Not only are these cages far too small, they normally have hard concrete floors which cause serious discomfort, as well as skin lesions. The chronic inactivity resulting from being penned up for most of their lives

---

[181] see Marchant-Forde (2009a).
[182] Fraser et al. (2013).
[183] Fraser et al. (2013).
[184] Broom and Fraser (2007); Fraser et al. (2013).
[185] Webster (2015).
[186] D'Eath and Turner (2009)

leads to an increased incidence of osteoporosis and arthritis in penned sows.[187] Given that farmers put sows in stalls to make the whole management process easier, it is ironic that one of the problems appears to be a reduction in the likelihood of a sow becoming pregnant. Stall-housed sows return to oestrus later than sows housed in groups.[188] However, sows housed in groups which suffer bullying from other sows may exhibit the same problem.

A summary of animal welfare science studies relevant to pig housing is set out elsewhere.[189] The results are clear that close confinement is not good for welfare. Sows kept in stalls often exhibit stereotyped behaviours and most of their natural behavioural needs are frustrated. A breeding sow will be kept for 2 years or thereabouts, after which she will be killed. The commonest reason for killing breeding sows is reproductive failure.[190]

In 2007, Karlen et al. (2007) of the Animal Welfare Science Centre in Melbourne published a study which was used successfully by Australian Pork Limited, the pig producer representative body, to support its claim that pregnant sows may without detriment be kept in sow stalls (cages not much bigger than the animal's body) for 6 weeks of any pregnancy. Karlen et al. showed no significant effect of sow stall versus group housing on cortisol, or productivity, while the levels of blood cells involved in the immune response were found to be within normal levels. The authors ignored their own observations, saying in the abstract 'there was a trend for higher...cortisol' in group-housed animals early in pregnancy, 'there were changes in some leucocyte sub-populations' and 'there was a trend...for a lower reproductive failure' in the stall-housed animals and the combination of reproductive

---

[187] Webster (2005).

[188] Broom and Fraser (2007); in order to get pregnant again after the birth of a litter of piglets, the sow must become sexually receptive and fertile again; this is 'oestrus'.

[189] Caulfield (2013).

[190] Hughes et al. (2010)

parameters resulted in sows housed in stalls weaning the equivalent of 39 more piglets per 100 mated sows (87). In other words, a series of results which did not exceed the threshold for statistical significance was transmuted into a result that every farmer would recognise – a claimed decrease in productivity unless pregnant sows were kept in stalls. The repeated reference in this work to statistical trends towards significant effect is arguably meaningless and misleading. Futhermore, note that this work was published, with these statements, in a reputable animal welfare science journal, *Applied Animal Behaviour Science*. Clearly, then, publication in a peer-reviewed journal is no guarantee of rigorous science.

It is apparent that good management of group housing systems can achieve good welfare, and indeed good productivity.[191] More recent work appears to suggest that giving pregnant sows housed in groups more space per sow may reduce the incidence of aggressive behaviour and (very) slightly decrease plasma cortisol. The effects were evident early after mixing sows in a new group, and were not seen a few days later. However, the authors observed that the experiment did not have sufficient precision to determine what is an adequate space allowance, while noting that 1.4 square metres per sow was 'too small'.[192]

The confinement of sows to farrowing crates (which are even smaller than sow stalls) after they have given birth continues to be a real welfare concern. The Senate Committee on Animal Welfare has recommended 'encouragement' of adoption of alternative approaches to farrowing crates to avoid welfare problems. However, the pig industry has vigorously defended the continued use of farrowing crates, on the basis they are necessary for the welfare of the piglets. As John Webster says, this is not a welfare argument, it is an economic argument.[193] The ostensible reason for putting sows into farrowing

---

[191] Caulfield (2013); Fraser et al. (2013).
[192] Hemsworth et al. (2013)
[193] Webster (2005).

crates is to prevent piglets being crushed by the sow. The sow is confined in a small area, separated by bars from its piglets, which are in the 'creep space'. Farrowing crates provide even less space than a sow stall; they only have to be 2.0 metres in length. There is science to show that, especially for pigs of increasing parity, crate dimensions are not sufficient to accommodate a sow lying on its side (it has to poke its legs through into an adjacent crate), or to get up and lie down without difficulty.[194]

Norway, Sweden and Switzerland have banned farrowing crates, and free farrowing systems are under development in countries such as Denmark and the Netherlands (the latter two being major pork producers).[195]

In 2007 the European Food Safety Authority produced a Scientific Opinion on welfare in pigs.[196] This extensive review noted:

- Housing of sows in farrowing crates severely restricts their freedom of movement which increases the risk of frustration. It does not allow them, for instance, to select a nest site, to show normal nest-building behaviour, to leave the nest site for eliminative behaviour or to select pen areas with a cool floor for thermoregulation.
- Sows' nest-building behaviour is triggered by internal hormonal factors...the motivation for nest building is high...as a consequence, lack of nesting material is very likely to cause stress and impaired welfare.
- The level of piglet welfare and mortality...remains a major problem.
- ...mortality due to crushing has been reported to be higher in loose housing systems.

---

[194] McGlone et al. (2004); O'Connell et al. (2007); Marchant-Forde (2009); Anil et al. (2002).
[195] Farm Animal Welfare Committee (2015) *Opinion on free farrowing systems.*
[196] Algers et al. (2007).

- In a recent large-scale study on indoor loose farrowing and crate systems, no difference in total piglet mortality was observed.
- It is the expert opinion of the working group that farrowing systems should allow for the handling of destructible nest material to enable investigation and manipulation activities.
- The ability for nest building should also take into consideration the welfare of the piglets.
- The use of loose farrowing systems should be implemented only if piglet mortality in them is no greater than the mean level of mortality where the sows are kept in non-loose farrowing systems.

The authors noted: *studies using larger sample sizes have shown that piglet mortality was the same whether the sow was crated or kept loose, or even that piglet mortality was lower in loose housing.* They referred to a study by Weber et al. in Switzerland, which analysed performance data concerning 44,837 farrowings, across 482 farms using crates, and 18,824 farrowings in 173 farms using loose farrowing systems. Total piglet mortality was 12.1% and the number of piglets weaned per sow mated was 9.6 (range about 0.02 for crates, 0.04 for loose), regardless of the system used.[197]

In 2010 the Australian pig industry (Australian Pork Limited), recognising public concerns about keeping pigs severely confined, published a review of farrowing systems by Dr Greg Cronin of the University of Sydney. Dr Cronin has extensive relevant experience in the area and has worked on APL-funded projects for many years. He was responsible for the development of the Werribee Farrowing Pen, which allows sows to move about, while protecting their young. The Cronin review acknowledged that keeping sows in a severely restricted space would thwart several behaviours which they are strongly motivated to perform (such as nest building). Cronin noted that prevention of nest

---

[197] Weber et al. (2007).

building and other associated behaviours would violate one of the 'Five Freedoms' in relation to animal welfare.[198]

The Cronin review rightly highlighted the consequences of moving away from a farrowing crate system for the pig farmer; the major economic impact (leaving aside any effect on productivity) would result from changes in stockperson skills resulting from having sows more able to move, plus probably changing the nature of flooring from slatted to solid, and providing bedding, probably in the form of straw. Obviously any additional space requirements would have cost implications.

The Cronin review is an extensive and competent summary of the relevant science to its publication date. It points out that the key parameter, so far as the farmer is concerned, is the number of piglets weaned per sow per litter. It notes, unsurprisingly, that the main cause of piglet death is crushing by the sow. Of 36 studies he reviewed, Cronin identified 64% which showed higher mortality in farrowing pens, compared to crates.

Weber and co-workers in Switzerland looked at piglet mortality in loose farrowing systems. They found that in 99 farms, with 12,155 farrowings, the average number of piglets weaned per sow mated was 9.7, with lower and upper quartiles of 8 and 11, respectively. The maximum was 16. This number can be compared with Australian data for 2011/2012, which showed that the average number of piglets weaned per sow mated was 9.88, with a minimum of 8.8 and a maximum of 11.65.[199] These data also show that the productivity in Sweden (which has banned farrowing crates; the rate is about 23.9 piglets per annum) is higher than Australia (23.0 piglets per annum)

---

[198] The 'Five Freedoms' were developed by the UK Animal Welfare Council, in response to the landmark Brambell Committee Report of 1965 into intensive farming practices.
[199] Australian Pork Limited *Australian Pig Annual 2012-13*.

There are obvious welfare benefits to the sow in not being restrained in a farrowing crate throughout the post-partum period until weaning.

It appears that both farm performance data and scientific studies indicate that comparable productivity (that is, piglets weaned per sow – reflecting total piglet mortality, including stillbirths) can be obtained in farrowing pens and farrowing crates. However, there may be some advantage to the piglets in confining sows for a few days after farrowing.

The overall conclusion is that present intensive systems for raising pigs are without doubt cruel and inhumane. They should be discontinued.

## Chickens

Broom and Fraser (2007) point out that chickens have a harder time of it than other farm animals because they are kept in such huge numbers, so are not thought of as individuals. They are also seen as very different from humans and other animals that humans feel well-disposed towards. There is a preconception that chickens, as birds, are not very clever (think 'bird brain'). However, this is not true.

It is likely that chickens exhibit a range of complex cognitive abilities. They can understand that an object still exists, even when out of sight, have a perception of time passing, have good memory skills, can use deductive reasoning to predict social interactions based on observing interactions between other individuals, and have complex communication abilities. They can recognise and discriminate many individuals within their own group and learn by observing others. It is thought they experience a range of positive and negative emotions.[200]

### Egg-laying chickens

In the absence of an independent scientific review as part of the process for development of an animal welfare code for chickens, RSPCA

---

[200] Marino (2016).

Australia has published its own review of layer hen welfare. This represents a valuable resource.[201]

Apart from the basic biological necessities, such as food, water and adequate living environment, chickens have a need to flap their wings, preen and dust-bathe, perch, explore and forage, interact with other chickens and have a nest for laying eggs. Laying hens in cages are adequately provided for in terms of nutrition, water and general environment, but are unable to express any of the natural behaviours referred to.[202] The restriction of movement and lack of perches in battery cages contributes significantly to a reduction in proper bone development, which results in up to 40% of laying hens (at end of lay) being found with broken bones.[203] Bone problems in egg-laying chickens are exacerbated by the high incidence of osteoporosis, seemingly because genetic selection for high rates of egg laying has led to excessive loss of bone calcium (which is repartitioned to egg shells).[204] Frustration of the birds' need to find a suitable nest site results in sterotyped pacing, while inadequate space for movement and separation from cage mates results in injurious pecking.[205]

In 1990 the Senate Committee on Animal Welfare recommended an end to battery cages be considered when viable alternative systems with welfare advantages were available.

---

[201] RSPCA Australia (2016).

[202] see Fraser et al. (2013); Nicol et al. (2017).

[203] Broom and Fraser (2007). The meta-analysis of Freire and Cowling (2013) also confirmed lower leg-bone strength in cage systems compared to other housing methods.

[204] Fraser et al. (2013).

[205] Broom and Fraser (2007). Note that Freire and Cowling (2013), reporting on a range of studies, did not find that aggressive pecking was worse in cage systems compared to other systems. Note also that 'aggressive pecking' may give a misleading impression; perhaps the more correct view is that this behaviour is 'redirected' ground pecking behaviour: Webster (2005); Nicol et al. (2017).

In 1996 the European Union Scientific Veterinary Committee reviewed the status of layer hen welfare.[206] Its conclusions included that hens strongly preferred to lay eggs in nests and were highly motivated to perform nesting behaviour. They also preferred littered flooring for pecking, scratching and dust-bathing. Hens preferred to perch, especially at night. The benefits of cage systems included separation of birds from manure, maintenance of small groups with a stable social order and low risk of cannibalism. The deficiencies of battery cage housing included restriction of natural behaviours, particularly nesting, perching and scratching, the prevalence of increased fear and bone weakness resulting from lack of movement. The Committee said 'it is clear that because of its small size and its barrenness, the battery cage as used at present has inherent severe disadvantages for the welfare of hens.' The Committee looked favourably on the use of enriched cages.

In 2005[207] the Scientific Advisory Panel of the EU reviewed the scientific literature and concluded that there were particular risks associated with keeping birds outdoors, citing incidence of disease as a concern. Injurious pecking was regarded as a problem and the Panel felt that it may spread more in a large flock of birds than in small groups. Bumble foot[208] was regarded as a problem in housing systems using perches. The Panel noted several studies demonstrating hens in furnished cages and non-cage (ie free range) systems have significantly stronger bone strength than hens housed in conventional cages. Handling and depopulation-induced bone breakage is lower in non-cage systems. Ammonia levels are usually higher in non-cage than in cage systems. Mortality rates were often higher in non-caged housing systems than in caged systems.[209]

---

[206] *The welfare of laying hens* (1996).

[207] Algers et al. (2005).

[208] Bacterial infection which causes extreme pain and Inflammation of the foot pad; it only appears in non cage systems or cage systems with perches.

[209] eg Elson (2015).

The 2005 Panel report made the following recommendations on housing-specific matters:

- All systems should provide sufficient space for walking and other activities;
- There should be genetic selection of birds destined for non-cage systems to minimise injurious pecking behaviour;
- Suitable nests should be provided;
- Facilities for foraging should be provided;
- Elevated perches should be provided;
- Beak trimming should be phased out, but only when suffering caused by cannibalism does not exceed that of the effects of the operation.

Another useful source of commentary on relevant science is the UK Farm Animal Welfare Council.[210] In 2007 the Council reported on welfare issues in the use of enriched cages. Referring to the LayWel project,[211] the Council noted the high mortality rates recorded in non-cage systems, but also pointed out that the final report from LayWel showed decreasing mortality rates in non-cage systems, compared with earlier findings; it speculated that this reflected improved management of the novel systems with experience. The LayWel project included the conclusion that 'with the exception of conventional cages, all systems have the potential to provide satisfactory welfare for laying hens.' It emphasised the restriction of natural behaviours by housing in conventional cages and the bone strength problems which occur in that system. FAWC concluded that well managed enriched cage systems are able to offer the potential for an acceptable balance between the requirements for a hen's health and welfare, and public health, in combination with economic and environmental considerations.

---

[210] Replaced by the Farm Animal Welfare Committee in April 2011: see http://www.defra.gov.au.

[211] A European Commission project to assess the implications of changes in production systems on laying hen welfare: see http://www.laywel.eu.

In 2010 the Council published an opinion on osteoporosis and bone fractures in laying hens. It remarked that bone weakness in laying hens mainly results from osteoporosis. Bone loss is decreased by load bearing and biomechanical forces (ie, as occurs during any sort of exercise). Bone loss is particularly likely with high egg production rates, as mobilisation of calcium for egg formation in effect redirects calcium from bone. It is very likely that bone fracture in laying hens is associated with severe and chronic pain. A large number of fractures occurred during depopulation of battery sheds. The Council's report regarded the level of bone fractures as increasing, and at an unacceptable level. An important recommendation was that industry should make serious efforts to reduce the rate of fractures. This should be coupled with proper monitoring.

A particularly important study is that of Sherwin and colleagues (of the University of Bristol), which analysed welfare indices in 26 commercial flocks, assessed at three points during the laying period. Observations were made on randomly selected focal hens in each flock. The study included observations of several novel welfare indicators, including egg calcification spots (said to be indicative of stress), egg blood stains and faecal corticosterone levels. The authors concluded that, overall, the welfare of birds was better in furnished cages than in the other housing systems. However, they cautioned that this seemingly positive outcome might reflect the 'novelty' of that housing system, which could be associated with application of better attention and diligence by the producers.

Another useful review is that of Lay et al.[212] These authors concluded that exposing hens to litter and soil in noncage and outdoor systems was associated with increased likelihood of disease and parasite infestation. Housing systems which limit movement, particularly conventional cage systems, are associated with osteoporosis, but there is evidence that providing increased complexity in housing systems (ie

---

[212] Lay et al. (2011).

in noncage systems) increases the incidence of bone fractures. Provision of more space allows for expression of a greater range of behaviours, but may also result in deleterious behaviours, such as cannibalism. Mortality can reach unacceptably high levels in noncage systems. An important point is that selective breeding for features such as improved bone strength and decreased feather pecking may provide significant welfare improvements. Overall, the authors' view was that no single housing system ranks high on all welfare parameters and no single breed of hen is perfectly adapted to all types of housing systems.

The most recent review of the literature is that of Nicol et al. (2017), commissioned by the Victorian government. This report was commissioned because of the failure of the industry-dominated review of the Poultry Standards and Guidelines to include an independent review of the relevant science. The review of Nicol et al. is a very comprehensive and careful review.

Free range systems have been criticised on various grounds, including that infections and parasites can be a problem if birds are not rotated to 'clean' areas sufficiently frequently. Several authors have reported that mortality is higher in free-range than other systems. Barrett et al. (2014) surveyed free range farm operators in the UK and found that many had experienced mortality due to smothering. They observed there were few effective strategies for reduction of smothering in free range flocks. Note, however, that Freire and Cowling (2013) carried out a meta-analysis of studies on layer hen welfare and found that mortality did not differ between the various housing systems. Nicol et al. (2017) remark on the higher incidence of mortality and smothering problems in non-cage systems.

The four types of layer hen housing system, that is conventional cages, non-cage indoor ('barn'), furnished cage and non-cage outdoor ('free range'), are each associated with positive and negative features regarding layer hen welfare. Conventional cage systems restrict expression of behaviour and are associated with increased incidence of bone weakness. On the plus side, conventional cage housing has been said to be associated with lower mortality and disease rates than non-cage systems. Furnished cages appear to offer welfare advantages on a range of measures. Complex housing environments, including free range, obviously allow greater expression of behaviour and choice, but may be associated with higher mortality – although Raf Freire's analysis disputes this (Freire and Cowling, 2013). The detailed review of the literature by Nicol et al. (2017) nevertheless shows that '...in a substantial minority of loose-housed flocks the levels of mortality can become extremely high', but goes on to note '...well-managed and designed free-range systems can produce low-mortality outcomes'.

I think the best conclusion is that the welfare disadvantages of conventional cage systems, that is the behavioural disadvantage, cannot be overcome, but the welfare disadvantages of non-cage systems can be overcome by good management practices.[213]

However, there is a further issue, which is that several studies have now shown that in free range systems, not all hens access the range daily; some hens never go outside;[214] even this is debatable, as a recent study using radio frequency identification technology showed that 70% to 80% of hens studied in two flocks accessed the range every day.[215] Clearly work must be done to further define the characteristics of the housing system and the range in order to create systems which encourage birds to go outside.

### Meat chickens (broilers)
The number of meat chickens in Australia has been increasing steadily for some considerable time; between 1965 and 2015, the number of

---

[213] See the proposal by Elson (2015), as an example.
[214] Pettersson et al. (2016); Campbell et al. (2016); see Nicol et al. (2017).
[215] Larsen et al. (2017).

birds slaughtered each year rose from about 50 million to nearly 630 million.[216]

Chicken meat production is a vertically integrated business. A handful of large companies control all aspects of production, from breeding establishments, feed mills, broiler growing farms and abattoirs.[217] In Australia, seventy percent of the industry is owned by two companies: Baiada and Inghams Enterprises. The activity of growing the chickens out is done by contract growers, of which there are about 800. The two main strains of meat chickens are the Ross (licensed from Aviagen to Ingham's) and the Cobb (licensed from Tyson Foods to Baiada Poultry).[218]

These animals have been selectively bred to achieve astonishingly high growth rates. They are killed at between 5 and 7 weeks of age, when they have reached a weight of up to 2kg. This amazing growth rate has negative consequences. As Broom and Fraser (2007) put it:

> '*the major fundamental problems of broiler production resulting in poor bird welfare are a consequence of selecting birds for a short, very fast-growing life. The birds will tend to be too heavy for normal locomotion and therefore develop leg disorders. Since leg disorders are disabling and often associated with inflammation of joints, hocks and bone, it is clear that their incidence may cause a major welfare problem...because lame broiler chickens are in pain when they walk.*'

Although there may be adequate room when young meat chickens are put into a shed, by the time they have reached killing weight they will be crowded. There can be up to 20,000 birds in one shed.[219] There is considerable accumulation of faeces, and the breakdown products are

---

[216] Australian Chicken Meat Federation: Industry facts and figures
www.chicken.org.au/page.php?id=4
[217] Australian Chicken Meat Federation www.chicken.org.au/page.php$ide=2.
[218] Robins and Phillips (2011).
[219] Broom and Fraser (2007).

corrosive to the skin, causing breastbone blister, hock-burns and footpad lesions. Elson (2015) has emphasised the need to maintain dry litter for meat chicken housing systems, whether intensive or otherwise. Wet litter is an important cause of contact dermatitis, which presents as foot pad dermatitis or hock burn. These conditions are very painful. There have been studies which have shown that foot pad dermatitis can in fact be much higher in free range (up to 98%) than intensive systems (average of 15%).[220] It is not clear why this should be so.

The rapid growth rate of the birds also has the consequence that the cardiovascular (heart, blood vessels) and pulmonary (lung) systems cannot cope with the circulatory and other demands of the muscles and gut. This failure causes build up of fluid in the abdominal cavity, known as ascites, which can be fatal.[221] The rapid growth of meat chickens requires feed restriction in order to prevent obesity and reproductive failure. The birds are therefore probably suffering chronic hunger.[222]

The major breeders have responded to the increased demand for free range meat from chickens by developing slower growing lines, such as Ross Rowan and Cobb Sasso. These birds take 50% to 100% longer to reach killing weights than the fast growth strains. The free range market in the European Union has also seen uptake of the French Label Rouge birds, which also grow more slowly.[223]

Stocking density, group size and shed size are obvious parameters which would be expected to influence welfare. However, as Robins and Phillips (2011) have pointed out, there are different welfare aspects affected at different stocking densities and 'no clear cut-off point at which welfare

---

[220] See Elson (2015).
[221] see Nicol et al. (2017).
[222] Fraser et al. (2013).
[223] Robins and Phillips (2011).

suddenly deteriorates'. There is evidence that providing meat chickens with straw bales has several positive effects on welfare.[224]

## Sheep

It now widely acknowledged that sheep feel pain like other animals, and methods for detecting and quantifying pain in sheep have become increasingly sophisticated.[225] Routinely, lambs are subjected to painful surgical interventions, including ear tagging, tail docking and castration. The excuse often given is that young sheep do not suffer pain as much as older animals. However, sheep are born with quite mature nervous systems and probably do not undergo significant nervous system development post-natally. The response to a painful thermal stimulus has been found not to differ between young and old sheep, although oddly, pain sensation was less in older male sheep, than female sheep.[226] Defending procedures such as mulesing on the grounds that pain perception is somehow different in sheep has no basis in scientific fact.

Broom and Fraser (2007) comment on the peculiarly Australian procedure of mulesing lambs. This involves catching the animal, holding it upside down in a frame, and slicing off a 15cm diameter area of skin. This is carried out primarily on Merino lambs. Mulesing is the cutting off of wrinkled skin around the perineum and anus of lambs, with resultant formation of smooth and scarred tissue. It is done to prevent urine and faecal soiling of the area, which in turn reduces flystrike. Flystrike occurs when blowflies lay eggs on the sheep and the hatched maggots feed on the affected area; it is a serious welfare problem.[227] Broom and Fraser (2007) observe that the mulesed lamb will usually make no sound, and walk away after the procedure, leading to those involved in the procedure forming the impression that the lamb feels no pain. This is

---

[224] see Robins and Phillips (2011).
[225] 'Researchers design AI system to diagnose pain levels in sheep': https://www.eurekalert.org/pub_releases/2017-05/uoc-rda053017.php
[226] Guesgen et al. (2011).
[227] Phillips (2009).

not true. Sheep have the anatomical and physiological bases for feeling pain. This includes relevant pain 'receptors' (nociceptors), pain transmitting nerve fibres, appropriate pain processing centres in the brain and spinal cord and pain-associated neurotransmitters.[228] Experiments have shown changes in mulesed lambs which indicate they experience pain after the procedure. The study of Paull et al. (2007) examined the pain-relieving effect of a local anaesthetic, lignocaine, alone or in combination with either carprofen or flunixin. These latter compounds are analgesics of the non-steroidal anti-inflammatory class. The authors made various behavioural measures indicative of pain, such as 'stiff walking' and 'hunched standing'; their data indicated that the most effective treatment was a combination of the local anaesthetic and carprofen. Using somewhat different behavioural measures of pain, Lomax et al. (2013) claimed that local anaesthetic alone was more effective than observed by Paull et al. (2007), and suggested that the local anaesthetic reduced mulesing pain for up to 24 hours after dosing. Windsor et al. (2016) have reported that over 40 million sheep have been treated with the registered local anaesthetic formulation Tri-Solfen since its introduction in 2005. 'as it clearly addresses pain and improves healing of mulesing wounds'. The claim that wound healing was improved with this formulation needs further study, in my view. Windsor et al. (2016) suggested that inclusion of a non-steroidal anti-inflammatory drug was a 'logical additional strategy'. In July 2016 the Australian Pesticides and Veterinary Medicines Association approved the use of the non-steroidal anti-inflammatory drug meloxicam for use in sheep and lambs.

In 2004, People for the Ethical Treatment of Animals (PETA) campaigned against the Australian sheep industry, claiming that mulesing was a barbaric and unnecessary practice.[229] PETA's action resulted in several clothing retailers refusing to use wool from mulesed sheep. Following an out of court settlement in the case of *Australian Wool Innovation Ltd*

---

[228] Broom and Fraser (2007).
[229] Sneddon and Rollin (2010).

*v Newkirk*,[230] the Australian wool industry undertook to phase out mulesing by 2010. That has not happened. In response to the outcry about mulesing, the Australian Wool Exchange (AWEX) in 2008 instigated the National Wool Declaration Integrity Program. This provides information to the prospective buyer about the mulesing status of wool batches, including whether the animals have received treatment with a registered product for pain relief.[231] A number of influential wool buyers have indicated they will not buy Australian wool from mulesed sheep (see Chapter 11).

## Cattle

The life of a dairy cow is very hard indeed. Selective breeding for very high milk production, at a high food conversion efficiency, itself imposes a great metabolic burden. There is good evidence that selection for increased milk yield is associated with a genetically-linked deterioration in overall fertility, occurrence of mastitis and lameness.[232] In modern dairy herds life expectancy for a cow can be as short as seven or eight years.

The misuse of science in the development of Australian Standards for animal welfare of cattle is illustrated by two recent examples: the time allowed for keeping bobby calves off feed, and the use of caustic paste for disbudding (removing horn buds) of calves.

### Bobby calves

Bobby calves are young unweaned mostly male dairy calves which are essentially by-products of the dairy industry. The Australian Animal Welfare Standards – Land Transport of Livestock notes that those involved in the development process did not reach an agreement on the allowable time that bobby calves could be kept off feed prior to

---

[230] Caulfield (2009).

[231] see www.awex.com.au/publications/national-wool-declaration-nwd/.

[232] See Webster (2005); Voiceless (2015) *The life of the dairy cow.*

slaughter; therefore the Standards are silent on the total time bobby calves can be kept off liquid feed (ie milk).

Phillips and Petherick (2015) have noted that there is a benefit to industry in having long allowable times off feed, as collection of calves from farms would be more economical. These authors have criticised the industry-funded research which has been used to support a voluntary industry code allowing bobby calves to be kept off feed for up to 30 hours (Fisher et al. 2014). The welfare measures in that work included various behaviours, changes in some blood metabolites (such as glucose), estimates of dehydration and change in weight. During 30 hours of food deprivation (which included transport periods), blood glucose fell substantially. As noted by Phillips and Petherick, while Fisher et al. maintained that the glucose levels recorded were within the normal published ranges for calves, 7 of the 60 calves studied had plasma glucose levels below normal ranges. Phillips and Petherick rightly point out that 'relying on group mean values may not be sufficient for welfare assessment, when individual animals may have impaired welfare'. They also note that even small reductions in blood glucose can produce feelings of hunger in humans; this suggests that the data of Fisher et al. may indicate that calves begin to feel hunger as soon as 3 hours after feeding. Fisher et al. concluded that 'the calves in the study coped with a period of 30 hours off feed but best practice would be represented by a period of not more than 24 hours'. Phillips and Petherick dismiss this, saying 'in our view welfare best practice would be no transport at all, i.e. slaughter on farm'. Finally, Phillips and Petherick criticise the use of 'reference ranges' of glucose, rather than the inclusion of an appropriate control group for comparison.

The Bobby Calf Regulatory Impact Statement, in considering the option of allowing a maximum of 24 hours time off feed (TOF), said 'there is no scientific evidence to suggest that 24hrs TOF provides any more additional animal welfare benefits than 30 hrs TOF...the ethical questions and value judgements of hypothetical animal 'hunger' and 'discomfort' are beyond the scope of the RIS...'. This is a misleading statement. As Phillips and Petherick point out, there were 'substantial changes in metabolite levels...particularly between 24 and 30 hours after feeding'.

The science considered in the development process for legislation governing bobby calf time off feed was therefore flawed, and the conclusions were unjustifiable.

### Removing horns

For many years farmers have taken steps to remove horns from cattle. One such step involves the application of caustic paste to dissolve the horn buds in young cattle. This paste contains very strong alkaline agents, such as sodium hydroxide or calcium hydroxide (Stafford and Mellor, 2011). These agents have been shown to cause pain when used for disbudding in calves.[233]

The existing Model Code of Practice for the Welfare of Animals: Cattle says that caustic paste should not be used for disbudding young calves. This prohibition is reversed in the endorsed Australian Animal Welfare Standards and Guidelines for Cattle (s. 6.5), which permits the use of caustic chemicals, without pain relief, for disbudding young calves (under 14 days of age). It has been claimed that this change was stimulated by recent scientific findings. Thus, there was a de-emphasis of the significance of a (relatively) early paper (Morisse et al. 1995), and emphasis on a study by Vickers et al. (2005). The Cattle Decision Regulation Impact Statement says, referring to Vickers et al., '...more recently, a study concluded that caustic paste causes pain, but that it is *less* than that caused by the hot iron, even when using local anaesthetic. Moreover, caustic disbudding has a lower impact in younger animals...Furthermore, chemical burns pain may be transient.'

All of these statements are false, for the following reasons:

---

[233] Morisse et al. (1995)' Vickers et al. (2005); Stilwell et al. (2009); Stilwell et al. (2010).

- Vickers et al. (2005) concluded that 'caustic paste dehorning with xylazine sedation (emphasis added) might be a more humane, simpler, and less invasive procedure than hot-iron dehorning with sedation and local anesthesia'; in other words, the paper supports caustic paste disbudding *with the use of xylazine*; all the calves in the study of Vickers et al. were pre-treated with xylazine 20 minutes before treatment with the paste. Xylazine is not only a sedative, but is also a powerful pain-killer (analgesic). It is therefore not surprising that caustic paste dehorning with xylazine may indeed be humane.

- The published evidence does not support the contention that the pain of caustic paste disbudding is less than that caused by use of the hot iron technique. The study of Morisse et al. (1995) found that caustic paste was more painful than hot-iron disbudding. Moreover, Stafford and Mellor (2011), in their review of the field, concluded that 'the cortisol response in the hours following cautery disbudding without anaesthesia or analgesia is lower than the response to chemical disbudding…which suggests that the former technique is less painful, acutely, than the latter [technique].' They go on to say 'chemical burns may be ongoing and deeper than the burns caused by cautery.'

- There is no evidence, either from the study of Vickers et al. (2005) or from other published science (which is not cited in the Cattle Decision Regulation Impact Statement), that 'caustic disbudding has a lower impact in younger animals'. Vickers et al. used animals aged 10-35 days, but did not remark on any lesser pain response in younger, versus older animals. Likewise, Stilwell et al. (2008) used animals in the range 10 to 40 days old and did not note any difference in pain response dependent on age of animal. Moreover, these authors found that an analgesic pre-treatment was quite ineffective in relieving the pain associated with the procedure. This argues against the description in the Cattle Decision Regulation Impact Statement of caustic paste pain as 'relatively low impact.' Stilwell et al. (2009) included animals in the age range alluded to in the Australian Animal Welfare Standards and Guidelines for Cattle standard relating to caustic paste use, and did not report any 'lower impact' of the procedure on the younger animals. Importantly, the study of Stilwell et al. (2009) showed that 'inert lying' was commonly seen in young calves treated with caustic paste, and they suggested this behaviour 'relates to the intense distress felt during the first few hours after the caustic burn'.

- The available evidence is that chemical burns pain is not 'transient'. Stilwell et al. (2009) cite references which describe human pain caused by caustic alkali as 'chronic'. It is entirely reasonable to assume that a calf will experience similar sensations after caustic paste disbudding. Stilwell et al. (2008) also noted elevated stress hormone levels in caustic paste-treated calves 3 hours after the treatment, and pain-related behaviours at 1 hour and 3 hours after treatment. The study of Vickers et al. observed pain-related behaviours in paste-treated calves for up to 4 hours after treatment; Stilwell et al. (2009) noted a high incidence of pain behaviours at 3 hours after the treatment. While the study of Morisse et al. (1995) did not detail pain behaviours at times less than 4 hours after treatment, their data do suggest that animals experience pain for at least 4 hours. The conclusion from these studies is that the pain of caustic paste disbudding in calves lasts for 3 hours and possibly more.

This shows how, when one drills down to the detail of the analysis in such government sponsored animal welfare code reviews, it is often the case that the science is misquoted and misrepresented, with conclusions being reached that suit the animal use industry. As I have shown, the scientific analysis relating to the pain of caustic paste disbudding in the Cattle Decision Regulation Impact Statement is selective in the papers it refers to, in that it does not refer to either the review of Stafford and Mellor, or the work by Stilwell et al., and furthermore the paper it does rely on (Vickers et al., 2005) is itself potentially flawed and in any case does not support the assertions made in the Statement.

A recent survey of Canadian and US farmers by Robbins et al. (2015) found that many farmers were against providing pain relief for dehorning and disbudding on the grounds not only of expense, but also because some believed the pain experienced was minimal and short lasting and in any case that pain control methods had little effect. In other words, they were ignorant of the facts. Robbins and colleagues note that pain relief can cost less than a cup of coffee and in any case pain relief can reduce the reduction in an animal's growth rate that occurs after dehorning.

## Australian animal welfare science today

In Australia, the study of animal welfare science for much of the last 50 years has been spent going round in circles, and we are still re-inventing the wheel. The UK Brambell Committee in 1965 started the ball rolling. It could be said to have laid the foundations for animal welfare science. It identified the problem areas, particularly in 'factory farming', and made practical suggestions about how to advance animal welfare. It leaned heavily on ethological and behavioural approaches and saw no problem with giving animals the 'benefit of the doubt'. It envisaged a committee made up of independent people, including scientists, to point the way forward. In 2005 Geoff Neumann and Associates (contracted by the Commonwealth Department of Agriculture) reviewed the state of the Model Codes of Practice for the Welfare of Animals. So, forty years after the Brambell Committee reported, Neumann noted: '...*international scrutiny has been mounting over a range of Australian animal husbandry practices with concern that the welfare outcomes from Codes do not provide assurance that the impact of some management practices is being addressed*'. He quoted Fraser's comments to the OIE, saying '*as animal management has become more intensive it has been perceived more as an industrial, technological and corporate activity resulting in a greater scrutiny of food production and a desire to see standards imposed'*. The Report advocated basing code reviews on an independent review of the relevant animal welfare science.

In Australia there has been virtually no progress more than ten years after the Neumann Report, and more than fifty years after Brambell. The current federal government's lack of interest in farm animal welfare is evidenced by the fact that the Neumann Report is nowhere to be found on any government website. Not only were the conclusions of the Neumann report ignored, but the federal government, in an act of vandalism, has made this important document disappear.[234] This means we are back where we were when the Brambell Report was produced.

As I have said, one of the important reasons to engage with animal welfare science is that scientific observations, done properly, are objective. This means that if the animal welfare scientist does his or her job correctly, the results will point in the right direction to improve animal welfare, with no emotionality or fuzzy warm feelings involved.[235] Professor Donald Broom summarised the position when he said in his and David Fraser's book on the subject: *'We pay tribute to...the late Ruth Harrison for drawing the attention of the world to farm animal welfare problems, and for frequent encouragement to Donald Broom and other welfare scientists to obtain precise evidence on matters relevant to welfare.'* (Broom and Fraser, 2007).

Those who use animals for profit scorn what they would describe as excessive anthropomorphism. So, the animal use industries, particularly those which keep animals in very close confinement, have repeatedly argued that the concerns of consumers may be more driven by emotional perceptions, rather than by any scientific rationale that a particular farming system, such as caging chickens or pregnant pigs, is

---

[234] Contrast this with the UK government approach, whereby all the reports (etc) of the Farm Animal Welfare Council are archived online.
[235] Broom and Fraser (2007).

detrimental to the welfare of those animals. The Senate Committee on Animal Welfare summarised the position in 1990, saying:

> *'Farmers...are concerned about inexperienced observers making judgements based on perceptions rather than knowledge. They are especially critical of arguments which rely on the attributions of human emotions and motive to animals. In short they are concerned that many of the concerns of critics are unfounded...'.*

This is still the position adopted by the animal use industries. For example, the egg industry representative body Australian Egg Corporation Limited recently described Hungry Jack's decision to stop using eggs from caged hens as 'driven by emotion and perception, not science or reality'. This sentiment reflects the statement some years ago by Andrew Spencer, the Chief Executive Officer of Australian Pork Limited that a decision by the Australian pig industry to voluntarily (partially) phase out sow stalls 'was not about animal welfare and there's no real science to the position held by consumers' (*sic*).[236] These sorts of statements echo the view expressed by scientists from Australia's leading animal welfare science group.[237] This represents a sort of scientific snobbery, put forward by those doing work which has been paid for by the industry, and is a view which the industry welcomes. As I have said earlier, the fact is that the sort of science these people are talking about is in many case highly questionable in any case.

The problem for the proponents of the crusade for 'science, not emotion' is that it is very likely that anthropomorphism is a completely inevitable consequence of the phylogenetic similarities between humans and non-human animals.[238] Most people have no problem acknowledging that animals experience pain and suffering. This is because they themselves know what pain and suffering is and can see that other species, being similar to them, will experience it. Despite this,

---

[236] See Caulfield (2013).
[237] Barnett et al. (2001).
[238] Westbury et al. (2011); Haynes (2011).

the development of animal welfare science, particularly regarding the attribution to animals of complex abilities and feelings, has been held back by anti-anthropomorphism. Significant numbers of scientists have been reluctant to even get involved with work addressing these questions, because 'they risked the scorn of other scientists and having difficulties in future in obtaining research funding and getting papers published'.[239]

The main scientific input concerning animal welfare matters in Australia comes at the point when lawmakers are considering revision of what were the animal welfare 'codes of practice', which, when revised, will have mandatory components which (the intention is) will then be picked up in the wording of regulations in the states and territories jurisdictions.

Things have changed little since the revision of the Pig Code[240] in 2005. At that time, the scientific input to the review was made by the firm of economic consultants who were running the process. The result was a travesty.[241] As things stand today, scientific input is chosen by industry representatives and ends up being biased in favour of the industry position.[242]

Funding for animal welfare science in Australia is more or less completely controlled by industry interests. Research funding from industry Research and Development Corporations is matched dollar for dollar by the Commonwealth Government. These Corporations include Meat and Livestock Australia, Dairy Australia, Australian Wool Innovation, the Australian Egg Corporation Limited and Australian Pork Limited.[243] The practical upshot of this is that many researchers who

---

[239] Broom (2014).
[240] *Model Code of Practice for the Welfare of Animals – Pigs (3rd edition)* 2007. See www.publish.csiro.au/book/5698/.
[241] See Caulfield and Cambridge (2008); Caulfield (2013).
[242] see Caulfield (2017).
[243] Goodfellow (2015).

might want to do work on animal welfare relating to farm animals must obtain funding from these industry bodies. In my opinion, arguably many of those who do get funding become captured by what their industry sponsors want.

Australia is still struggling to escape a scientific viewpoint of animal welfare which is completely focused on physical health and biological functioning of animals, while devaluing aspects such as carrying out natural behaviours, or exhibiting abnormal behaviours. The dominant group for many years has been the Melbourne-based Animal Welfare Science Centre, led by Professor Paul Hemsworth. This group has promoted the view that 'fitness', as measured (for example) by reproductive performance is 'useful to the welfare debate' because of the direct and indirect detrimental consquences that physiological responses that are of a sufficient magnitude to detrimentally affect growth, reproduction or health reduce 'fitness'. They have said 'there is little evidence that behavioural change…is associated with a reduction in 'fitness'.' This group has relentlessly pushed the measurement of adrenocortical hormones (so-called stress hormones) and other biochemical and blood measurements as truly indicative of an animal's welfare state. They have said that aberrant behaviours, such as sterotypies, 'may be regarded as a mechanism that helps animals to cope with environmental change'. I interpose that a non-scientific view of this idea is that if you break your leg, you may alleviate the distress you feel by banging your head against the wall. Finally, they have said that there is great difficulty in using measurement of abnormal behaviours to assess welfare.[244] Much of the funding for this group's work has come from industry.

Eminent animal welfare scientist John Webster has characterised the Australian position thus:[245]

---

[244] Barnett and Hemsworth (1990).
[245] Webster (2005).

*'When scientists in the European Community and Australia were asked to review the welfare of sows in pregnancy stalls, the Australians concluded that confinement stalls for pregnant sows were acceptable on welfare grounds; the Europeans concluded that they were not. The two groups had studied the same evidence but apportioned value differently. According to the Australian view, the sows in confinement stalls showed an acceptable degree of fitness and this was sufficient reason to justify the system on the grounds of animal welfare. The European view was that the denial of natural behaviour was sufficient reason to impose a ban. While fitness is an essential element of good welfare, <u>it is not a sufficient description of good welfare</u> (emphasis added).'*

The position of these influential Australian scientists has, in my view, resulted in many negative consequences for farm animals in this country.

## Some current animal welfare frameworks

As we move towards a situation where some practical measures might be needed to assess whether farmers are using practices which provide acceptable levels of animal welfare, it is necessary to have schemes which can be applied to audit those practices.

The 'Five Freedoms' have been widely quoted and are rightly recognised as having served a useful purpose in focusing people's minds on how to improve farm animal welfare. They are all outcome measures, which direct readers to husbandry strategies necessary to promote the stated outcomes. They (arguably) do not embrace the concept of positive welfare states.[246]

Broom's definition of animal welfare (taking into account how an animal is coping with a situation) has gained wide acceptance in the animal welfare science community and elsewhere. For example, the World

---

[246] See Webster (2016).

Organisation for Animal Health (or OIE) repeats Broom's concept of 'coping', then expands on it; it has defined animal welfare as:

> '...how an animal is coping with the conditions in which it lives. An animal is in a good state of welfare if (as indicated by scientific evidence) it is healthy, comfortable, well nourished, safe, able to express innate behaviour, and if it is not suffering from unpleasant states such as pain, fear, and distress. Good animal welfare requires disease prevention and veterinary treatment, appropriate shelter, management, nutrition, humane handling and humane slaughter/killing/ Animal welfare refers to the state of the animal; the treatment that an animal receives is covered by other terms such as animal care, animal husbandry and humane treatment'.[247]

So this takes Broom's definition, which is useful to an animal welfare scientist, and tacks on to it some indications of what might be done to improve or maintain welfare.

In 2012 the World Organisation for Animal Health adopted 10 'General Principles for the Welfare of Animals in Livestock Production Systems'.[248] These are:

- genetic selection should always take into account the health and welfare of animals;
- the physical environment including the substrate (walking surface, resting surface etc) should be suited to the species and breed so as to minimise risk of injury and transmission of diseases or parasites to animals;
- the physical environment should allow comfortable resting, safe and comfortable movements, including normal postural changes, and the opportunity to perform types of natural behaviour that animals are motivated to perform;

---

[247] from the Terrestrial Animal Health Code: www,oie,int/doc/ged/D5517.pdf.
[248] Fraser et al. (2013).

- social grouping of animals should be managed to allow positive social behaviour and minimise injury, distress and chronic fear;
- air quality, temperature and humidity in confined spaces should support good animal health and not be aversive to animals. Where extreme conditions occur, animals should not be prevented from using their natural methods of thermoregulation;
- animals should have access to sufficient feed and water, suited to the animals' age and needs, to maintain normal health and productivity and to prevent prolonged hunger, thirst, malnutrition or dehydration;
- diseases and parasites should be prevented and controlled as much as possible through good management practices. Animals with serious health problems should be isolated and treated promptly or killed humanely if treatment is not feasible or recovery is unlikely;
- where painful procedures cannot be avoided, the resulting pain should be managed to the extent that available methods allow;
- the handling of animals should foster a positive relationship between humans and animals and should not cause injury, panic, lasting fear or avoidable stress;
- owners and handlers should have sufficient skill and knowledge to ensure that animals are treated in accordance with these principles.

Mellor (2016a) has recently re-focused on the Five Freedoms and the limitation that their primary focus is on preventing an animal undergoing negative experiences. He says this is not adequate, given the increasing recognition that animals may experience positive emotional states, which can be promoted (see also Sandoe and Jensen, 2011; Mellor 2016b). He also notes that the negative experiences referred to in the Five Freedoms cannot in effect be eliminated, because they are part of normal behaviours essential for survival, such as thirst and hunger. He identifies 'Animal Welfare Aims':

- Minimise thirst and hunger and enable eating to be a pleasurable experience.
- Minimise discomfort and exposure and promote thermal, physical and other comforts.
- Minimise breathlessness, nausea, pain and other aversive experiences and promote the pleasures of robustness, vigour, strength and well-coordinated physical activity.
- Minimise threats and unpleasant restrictions on behaviour and promote engagement in rewarding practices.
- Promote various forms of comfort, pleasure, interest, confidence and a sense of control.

He regards these as consistent with some of the aims of the European Welfare Quality assessment system for livestock, and also draws parallels with his Five Domains Model for animal welfare assessment, which he originally developed in 1994 (see Mellor and Beausoleil, 2015). Webster (2016) in assessing some of the various schemes, notes that the Five Domains model seeks to assess the impact of the environment (in its broadest sense) on the mental state of the animal; he contrasts this with the Five Freedoms (as qualified with the five provisions), which is outcomes-based. He sees the Domains model as having utility for scientists as a foundation for research and evidence based conclusions regarding impact on the mental state of animals.

The Welfare Quality project recognised that consumer perception of food quality was determined not only by overall nature and safety but also by the welfare status of the animals involved.[249] The project operates under four major headings (good feeding, good housing, good health and appropriate behaviour), which are further broken down into welfare criteria. A major thrust of the project is to move away from assessments based on observations of the environment, and to move more towards animal-based measures.[250] This is really very important,

---

[249] Blokhuis (2008).
[250] see Vapnek and Chapman (2010).

as many assessment schemes occupy themselves too much with things other than assessing the welfare state of the animal.[251]

All of this moves towards a view that animal welfare assessment can usefully be based on looking at the 'quality of life' of an animal.[252] This is aligned with the ideas of 'a life worth living' developed by the UK Farm Animal Welfare Council.[253] Such schemes would necessarily aim to devise codes of practice which included elements aimed at improving positive experiences. Useful moves towards achieving this would include giving serious consideration to characterising possible positive affects.

Mellor (2016b) has also noted that reference to the Five Freedoms has become something of an unthinking mantra used by some animal advocacy groups (and others), the implication being that they are fully achievable. As he says, this may be because they are couched in easily recognisable terms. The original Five Freedoms, as set out by John Webster, were never intended to represent the ideal, nor some absolute standard representing the pinnacle of good animal welfare. The intention was rather they were a checklist which could be applied to compare different systems. As Webster says, they are intended as no more than a memorable set of signposts to right action. Indeed, the very use of the word 'freedom' creates a set of conditions, which if taken literally, are unattainable in any farming setting. The emphasis should rather be on managing things so that negative experiences (for example) can be kept within tolerable limits.[254]

The Five Freedoms and their associated 'provisions' have undoubtedly achieved much, especially in the UK. I don't think there is much to be gained by sniping about whether or not they represent a perfect formulation. The fact is they moved things forward appreciably in the

---

[251] Webster (2005).
[252] see Green and Mellor (2011).
[253] see Sandoe and Jensen (2011); Webster (2016).
[254] Webster (2005); (2016).

UK. In fact, in Australia, if governments and industry paid any attention to what the Five Freedoms said, there would be huge advances. The likelihood of that happening in the foreseeable future is, in my view, minimal.

While these ideas and schemes are laudable, I think there is still a very long journey to be made to really implementing them. When one looks at what is actually going on daily in the animal use industries, it is very apparent that the sort of concepts being talked about are a long way from reality. For example, most of the aims referred to in any of the schemes referred to are not achieved when you keep hens in battery cages. Moreover, there is the overlying problem of trying to weigh up one welfare measure against another. Welfare can never be assessed as the algebraic sum of measures, some in one direction and some in the other. Taking the example given by Webster (2016), in the case of a dairy cow, can one quantify the extent to which 'affectionate sociability' can offset the pain of chronic lameness? In fact, Rollin (2015) has it right when he says that one's 'concept of welfare determines what counts as sound science'. This is the corollary of saying that the weight given to one welfare measure as opposed to another is imponderable. If one takes the view that a productive animal is in a good state of welfare, there will be less concern over issues such as the animal's mental state. Conversely, an attitude which *a priori* focuses on the overall wellbeing of the animal will necessarily take into account how it is feeling. What this means, in effect, is we will be going around in circles for some considerable time if we rely on science to resolve what is essentially an ethical dilemma. It also means that scientists engaged in this area must acknowledge that their work does not go on in an ethical vacuum, and they must accept the ethical consequences of what they do and what they find.

## Conclusions

Unfortunately, a great deal of Australian animal welfare science is, in my view, second-rate. The obsession with 'physiological' measures, and the de-emphasis of behavioural and other measures, has resulted in an over-interpretation of data which I suggest would not happen in the realm of physiological science. Too often one sees minute changes in 'stress hormones' interpreted as indicative of poor welfare, or worse still, lack of detectable changes in hormones as indicating that animals are in a good state of welfare. Nowhere is this more evident than where animals are put in extreme confinement, such as sow stalls for pregnant pigs, or battery cages for chickens. An endocrinologist, clinical veterinary scientist or physiologist looking at these data would dismiss them as meaningless. People working in those sorts of disciplines would attribute meaning only to changes which really mean something to the animal, as for example with Cushing's disease, where there is very significant elevation of adrenocortical hormone secretion. The piddling flickers of changes in levels seen in animal welfare science studies would be regarded as little more than background noise. In any case, they completely ignore the high level of complexity which is probably the reality of signalling between the brain and the point of hormone secretion. Somehow one is expected to believe that the mental state of an animal is reflected in a tiny increase or decrease of a hormone, maintained at that level for lengthy periods of time. This ignores the reality. To make matters worse, much of this poor animal welfare science is exacerbated by inappropriate use of statistics. Where no change is seen, according to the statistical threshold chosen by the scientists themselves, the experimenters, who are determined to see a change, spin the statistics and bend the results to claim significant effects where there are none. The game of spin continues with behavioural studies, where it is often said that choice experiments are the best way of showing what an animal's true preferences are. But even this is done in a cynical way, as to my knowledge none of the scientists concerned have done the obvious experiment of opening the cage to see what the animal does. I am sure most would agree that the likeliest choice is the animal leaves the cage; it most certainly will not return to spend the rest of its life there. Indeed, this hardly needs science; it is common sense. Unsurprisingly, this stuff is paid for by industry.

# Chapter 5    The law relating to animals

In 1964, Ruth Harrison presciently said: '*...if one person is unkind to an animal it is considered to be cruelty, but where a lot of people are unkind to a lot of animals, especially in the name of commerce, the cruelty is condoned and, once large sums of money are at stake, will be defended to the last by otherwise intelligent people'*. That summarises the problem which still exists today.

Writing about animal law in Australia is difficult, because (as set out below) most of the relevant offences must either be dealt with by a lower court (eg a Local Court or Magistrates Court), or can be dealt with by such a court if all parties agree. This is because the penalties for the offences concerned do not cross the threshold such that the cases have to be heard in a Supreme Court. There are one or two exceptions relating to serious aggravated cruelty, and these are dealt with below. However, the upshot of this is most animal cruelty and animal welfare cases go unreported in the legal publications or databases. Also, there are very few appeals from the decisions of the lower courts to courts whose decisions are reported.

## Early legislation

It seems that the first law seeking to protect animals from cruelty was enacted by the colony of Massachusetts Bay in 1641. It prohibited 'Tirrany or Crueltie' towards 'bruite Creature[s]'.[255] But this really was well ahead of its time. In England, for example, brutality towards animals, and the torture of animals as entertainment was commonplace. The ruling class had hunting, while the lower classes enjoyed 'sports' such as cock fighting and bull-baiting. Indeed, there is good evidence that blood sports were regarded as 'refined pleasures'.

Until the end of the eighteenth century, the legal treatment of animals was to regard them exclusively as forms of property, whereby the only rights involved were the rights of their owners. So, poaching in a royal

---

[255] See Singer (1975), 303.

forest was an offence punishable by death, and interfering with another person's cattle was punishable by a fine payable to the owner.

During the eighteenth century the generalized culture of violence, which hitherto had been associated with manliness and strength, began to be criticised. Hogarth's *Four Stages of Cruelty*, produced in 1751, literally illustrated the negative aspects of cruelty to animals. There emerged from the aristocratic classes a concept of the honour of being virtuous, and from that the idea that a gentleman had no truck with barbarity. One of the factors which contributed substantially to the development of concern for animals in London was the driving of cattle and sheep through London streets to the Smithfield market, and its attendant slaughterhouses, on the eastern side of London. The evolution of London, with the business district in the City area (very close to the market) and the fashionable West End nearby, meant the cruelty inflicted on these animals was very much in the face of Londoners.[256]

In 1800 a bill was introduced to the House of Commons to prohibit the sport of bull-baiting. Its sponsor, Sir William Pulteney, emphasised that the 'sport' was one engaged in by the lower classes, and in drawing together 'idle and disorderly persons' was often a stimulus for 'mischievous proceedings'.[257] It is interesting to note that another MP, social campaigner William Wilberforce, was displeased that Pulteney did not emphasise the cruelty aspect more. The Bill was ridiculed, and failed. One of the main lines of attack was that it sought to interfere with people's freedom to choose what they wanted to do. But as a generality, those that promoted the idea of better treatment of animals were widely regarded as lunatics. Another similar Bill, introduced in 1802, also failed. In both these cases, many Members of the House gave speeches extolling the virtues of these spectacles. Notably, nobody

---

[256] Kean (1998). She points out the irony of there being proper regulations regarding slaughter at that time in the 'infant colony' of New South Wales.
[257] See Radford (2001).

wanted to discuss the blood sports of the upper classes, such as fox hunting.[258]

In 1809, Lord Erskine introduced a Bill into the House of Lords seeking to protect cattle and horses from mistreatment. His main argument for it related to the intrinsic moral value of animals; indeed he referred to the God-bestowed moral trust which was a corollary of Man's dominion over animals. Although the Bill passed in the Lords, it was lost in the Commons by 10 votes. Regardless, it was widely reported in newspapers of the time and was generally well-received.

In 1821, Richard Martin, the member for Galway, introduced a bill seeking to protect horses. One has to remember this was in the context of a time where horses were the main mode of transport and source of power, expanding greatly with the industrial revolution. In the early 1800s in England there were over half a million horses employed outside agriculture. Abuse of horses will have been an everyday spectacle.[259] Martin's Bill suffered the same fate as its predecessors. However, an *Act to Prevent the Cruel and Improper Treatment of Cattle* was passed in 1822. In the following four years, Martin introduced nine further bills, all of which failed. And right up to that point, and afterwards, the idea of legislation to protect dogs was laughed at. In large part this was because pets were regarded as very much private property.[260]

Martin and colleagues, including William Wilberforce, went on to establish the Society for Prevention of Cruelty to Animals. This played the major role in enforcing the new law, as at the time there was no police force as such. According to Mike Radford, the society successfully prosecuted 149 cases of cruelty in its first year. The fortunes of the SPCA, at first precarious, improved steadily and in 1835 the then Princess Victoria became a patron. After becoming Monarch she

---

[258] Bargheer (2006).
[259] Kean (1998); Bargheer (2006).
[260] Kean (1998).

allowed it to use the prefix 'Royal'. She remained an ardent supporter; in 1887, for example, she referred to the 'growth of more humane feelings towards the lower animals' as a 'mark of the spread of enlightenment amongst my subjects'.[261]

The legislation continued to develop, with an Act in 1849 which made it an offence to 'cruelly beat, ill-treat, over-drive, abuse or torture any animal'. The significance of this was that the prosecution no longer had to establish that the cruelty was 'wanton'. This is important, as it is notoriously difficult to establish intention. Also the term 'animal' was defined, with the important inclusion at the end of 'any other domestic animal'. A later Act (1854) clarified the definition to include 'any other kind or species whatever and whether a quadruped or not', which effectively brought birds under the protection of the law. Importantly, the Act included a provision which made it an offence to transport an animal in a way that 'caused it unnecessary pain or suffering'. This was very different from the earlier acts, which were based on a list of proscribed practices; for the first time it introduced something like a general cruelty offence.

The first half of the nineteenth century was also characterised by a sustained attack maintained by the RSPCA and its parliamentary supporters on all of the then-prevailing cruel sports, such as dog fighting, cock fighting, bull running and so on.[262]

## Modern legislation

Early Australian legislation was based on the English animal protection law. The first such act was passed in Tasmania in 1837, followed by New South Wales (1850). then the four remaining colonies (by 1860).[263] The forerunner of much modern legislation, including Australian legislation, was the UK *Protection of Animals Act 1911*. It became an offence to 'cruelly...beat, kick, ill-treat, override, over-drive, overload, torture,

---

[261] Bargheer (2006).
[262] Harrison (1973).
[263] Goodfellow (2015).

infuriate, or terrify any domestic or captive animal, or wantonly or unreasonably to do or omit to do any act which caused such an animal unnecessary suffering'. Despite this, Radford (2001) notes that interest in helping animals stagnated for several decades during and after the two World Wars; there was not really a resurgence of activity until the 1960s. Arguably things moved much more slowly in Australia.

When considering an ethical framework for modern law relating to animal welfare, and animal cruelty, it is useful to not only think about not mistreating animals, but also to think about imposing a duty to look after animals. This latter approach would seem to fit with the 'guardianship' construct of Tischler (1977), and the feminist-inspired ethic of care.[264] Another point well made by Ruth Abbey (referring to Roger Scruton's work) is that different classes of animals may need to be treated differently. For example, pets and wild animals need to be considered differently when formulating any duties they may be owed.[265]

There are those who persist in saying (as was said from the early 1820s) that legislation is not needed, and that market forces will serve as an adequate expression of the views of the community. I agree with Mike Radford's contrary view that society's perceived collective values, in this instance, need to be reflected through legal regulation.[266] The morality of the market (if it has any) is not that of the community.

As is the case in the UK, Australian law is premised on utilitarian principles. There is also a faint argument that at least some of the law is based on respect for the intrinsic value of animals.[267] In Australian (and UK) jurisdictions, the core concept is that cruelty is not permitted, except where that cruelty is necessary and reasonable.[268] Therein is the

---

[264] Albright (2002).
[265] Abbey (2007).
[266] Radford (2001).
[267] see for example Webster (2005).
[268] see Bloom (2008).

rub; the reality is that the interests of the animal are made secondary to the interests of people, despite the often trivial nature of these latter interests.

As an aside, it is worth observing that guidance for the formation and evolution of Australian law must necessarily come from a limited number of similar jurisdictions – primarily the UK, the European Union and New Zealand, if only because there is so much divergence between nations regarding animal welfare legislation. For example, in the USA, farm animals are virtually exempt from animal welfare legislation. Many countries still have no animal welfare laws at all, and many of those that do have no interest in enforcement.[269]

## Regulation of animal welfare

Timoshanko (2015) notes that there are three broad categories of regulation: 'a binding set of rules to be applied by a body devoted to the purpose', 'any deliberate state influence in business or social affairs' and 'any form of social or economic influence'. Aspects of animal welfare in Australia are arguably regulated in all of these ways.

Reflecting the evolution of animal welfare laws from those dealing with cruelty to those also dealing with 'welfare', it will be seen that current laws have 'negative' aspects, prohibiting certain sorts of behaviour, and 'positive' aspects, in essence reflecting the imposition of certain duties.[270]

The challenge for those considering the regulation of animal welfare is the same as for those thinking about making laws to protect very young children or people with severe intellectual impairment. The subjects requiring protection cannot speak for themselves. While this is a statement of the obvious, the design of a regulatory system to look after animal welfare must take this into account. This can be dealt with easily enough where egregious cruelty to animals is involved, as authorised

---

[269] See White (2013).
[270] Timoshanko (2015).

officers can be put in a position where evidence can be gathered and prosecutions started. But the situation is very different in that, as Bloom (2008) has said, 'much animal welfare regulation must rely on the substantial voluntary compliance of those regulated'. This especially applies to animal use industries, particularly farming. Farmers will simply engage in disobedience of the law if attempts are made to criminalise what they see as normal acceptable behaviour regarding their treatment of animals. That means where there is a disconnection between what the society at large wants, and what the farmers do, a means must be found to reconcile that and achieve an improvement in practices. This requires not only the threat of sanctions, but a positive engagement of farming organisations to encourage adoption of welfare-friendly techniques.

I think there is sufficient and growing community interest in protecting the welfare of animals to continue to push for improvements in the way animal welfare is regulated.[271] Conversely, I consider it is unlikely that significant improvement in animal welfare will be achieved solely by leaving it to economic or market forces. While some improvements can be made by, for example, the response of the major supermarkets to consumer concerns, that will not be sufficient to address all animal welfare issues. It is also true, however, that there is a multi-tiered system of animal welfare regulation, premised on the visibility of the animals concerned. Where there is a lack of visibility, as is the case with farm animals, and particularly so with those using intensive housing systems, then the reality of their treatment is hidden from the public. The result is that they are not given equal consideration with, for example, companion animals, which are highly visible.[272]

As I have already mentioned, it is clear that animal welfare science can have a very important role in improving animal welfare.[273] Bloom (2008)

---

[271] See Bloom (2008).
[272] O'Sullivan (2012).
[273] see Chapter 4.

notes the useful role which science can play in formulating laws to improve animal welfare. He echoes Radford (2001) in pointing out that developing laws only on the basis of established science 'runs the risk of making animals the default victims of the current state of our knowledge or ignorance'. This is an important point. Science is there to inform and guide, not to rigidly define. There is every reason, as indicated by the Brambell Committee, for exercising the precautionary principle and giving animals the benefit of the doubt. On the other side of this coin, the farming lobby routinely uses science as an excuse for doing nothing to improve the lot of animals, which of course is their preferred position. Or worse still, they promulgate what I would describe as 'fake science' to support the *status quo*. As described in chapter 4, this is exemplified by the strong emphasis on studies of 'stress hormones', which invariably give the result farmers prefer, that is that their practices, particularly intensive housing in cages or stalls, do not cause animals stress.

Regulation of animal welfare involves many other interests apart from those directly relevant to the animals themselves. The most obvious examples include economic considerations, the environment, planning matters, health concerns, food safety and quality, tourism and entertainment (Bloom, 2008).

Australian jurisdictions are some considerable way behind Europe in terms of approaches to developing animal welfare legislation. In Australia, key provisions, especially relating to farm animals, are developed by committees, panels and the like which are dominated by industry interests. Scientific reviews are not carried out by independent scientists, but are instead done by economic consultants.[274] Close examination of these exercises again reveals the dominant influence of industry. The science is heavily selected and arguably biased. Moreover, Australian politicians involved in this area have a habit of engaging in

---

[274] See Caulfield and Cambridge (2008); Caulfield (2017). See also RSPCA Australia (2016).

'gesture politics'; they are very keen to demonstrate their concern for animal welfare, but are in actuality unwilling to make the hard decisions. Where they have made the hard decisions, the backlash from industry interests has often been enough to drive them out of office. The recent example of New South Wales Premier Mike Baird and his failure to stop greyhound racing, at the cost of his political career, is a case in point.

Australian governments regularly self-award themselves the status as 'world leaders' in animal welfare practices.[275] Any sensible person will see this is as embarrassing puffery. Indeed, World Animal Protection's Animal Protection Index reveals that this sort of claim is totally without foundation. It uses criteria designed to assess the quality of a country's animal protection laws. It rates Australia as a 'C', along with France, Spain, Brazil, Phillipines, Italy, Poland and Malaysia. Austria, Switzerland, the United Kingdom and New Zealand get an 'A' rating, while Denmark, Netherlands, Chile, Germany and Sweden get 'B'.[276] So by that rating, Australia is some considerable way from 'leading the world'.

Contrast this with the arrangements in Europe, where the European Union (though the European Commission) routinely uses committees composed of independent experts to advise on animal welfare matters. One such influential committee was the Scientific Veterinary Committee (Animal Welfare Section); its modern equivalent is the European Food Safety Authority Scientific Panel on Animal Health and Welfare Legislation.[277]

A further difficulty arises from the fact that Australia lacks a strategy for dealing with animal welfare. The European Union, for example, has developed the European Union Strategy for the Protection and Welfare

---

[275] See for example the website of the Department of Agriculture and Water Resources at www.agriculture.gov.au/animal/welfare/export-trade.
[276] www.worldanimalprotection.org.
[277] Broom (2009).

of Animals 2012-2015. As that strategy notes, it deals with issues relating to the 'keeping of billions of animals for economic purposes'. The EU Strategy notes that there is ongoing lack of enforcement of relevant rules, that consumers still need more education on animal welfare issues, and there is a need to simplify and develop clear principles for animal welfare. Australia is nowhere near achieving anything in this regard.

The options available to lawmakers concerning improvements in animal welfare are basically twofold. They can impose legal requirements (so-called 'command and control' or 'punish and deter') or they can engage in cooperation with industry, emphasising a remedial approach to unsatisfactory practices (the 'deterrence' approach).[278]

Goodfellow (2015) expresses the view that the enforcement approach to regulating animal treatment in the 'domestic realm' (ie companion animals, etc) is deterrence-oriented, while the approach where agricultural animals is concerned tends to be much more compliance based. Indeed, the regulation regarding domestic animals is primarily in the anti-cruelty and animal welfare statutes, while regulation of agricultural animals is to be found in subordinate legislation made under those acts.

The difficulties of a 'command and control' strategy are obvious. Not only does this sour the relationship between the regulators and the regulated, it also runs the risk of failure when brought to a court or tribunal, as well as inevitably involving serious expenditure. As Geoff Bloom says 'cooperation is usually cheaper and better than punishment'. That said, the threat of punishment should be ever-present.

I tend to agree with Bloom's suggestion that there should be two sets of statutes: one which deals with egregious cruelty, and another set which is more administrative in nature and regulates compliance with

---

[278] See Bloom (2008); Goodfellow (2015).

standards (and that would involve mostly animals in agriculture). I also agree with his suggestion that a licensing system, with appropriate licence conditions designed to maximise animal welfare, could be an approach which might work for agricultural animals. However, regardless of the approach, and no matter how much enforcer-user cooperation there is, nothing will work unless the enforcer is in a position to make unannounced inspections, with sanctions available in the event there has been failure to comply with the relevant law.

Industry often espouses the use of 'co-regulation' in relation to animal welfare. Bloom (2008) says that 'co-regulation empowers those subject to regulation to find the most appropriate ways for their activities to be performed in compliance with the required operational outcomes and standards that government...sets'. The current Exporter Supply Chain Assurance Scheme which seeks to set animal welfare standards for the treatment by importing countries of exported Australian animals is an example of such an arrangement.[279] However, the difficulty with co-regulation to assure animal welfare standards are maintained arises when one considers how to monitor whether standards are being complied with. The 'snapshot' approach of inspection at a particular time by a government officer may not be sufficient to ensure the welfare of all animals concerned is maintained at all times.[280]

Another approach which is commonly adopted by governments to regulation of challenging animal welfare problems is to do nothing. This is premised on the idea that the market will serve as the ultimate regulator. If consumers don't like something, for instance that an egg on a supermarket shelf is laid by a chicken in a battery cage, they won't buy it, so the argument goes. Timoshanko (2015) presents a cogent criticism of reliance on market forces to regulate animal welfare. He notes that price is a very significant limitation on a consumer's ability to choose high welfare products. A consumer may not want to buy eggs

---

[279] Chapter 7.
[280] Bloom (2008).

produced under cruel conditions, but may not be able to afford the premium which has to be paid for free range eggs. In support of this point, Timoshanko points to a survey by Coles which indicates that almost all consumers would switch to free range eggs were the price lower. However, surveys suffer from the problem that people do not always do what they say they will do. It is instructive to ponder what people would actually do if cage eggs were no longer available. Would they not buy eggs at all? Or would the relatively small increase in price which would be associated with a move to free range eggs result in the extra cost to the consumer being accepted?

These somewhat theoretical considerations are probably largely irrelevant given what is happening in practical terms. The development of animal welfare regulation in Australia is in a state of crisis. Since the attempt (starting in about 2005) to develop a country-wide standardised approach to the question, the various proponents on either side of the argument (that is, the farmers, versus the animal protection and welfare groups) have moved further and further apart. The battle is being won by the farmers. In the recent Productivity Commission report into regulatory burden in the farming sector, animal welfare was not raised as a concern by the farming lobby groups. One can only surmise that they have in effect neutralised the threat which the emerging power of the animal protection groups presented several years ago. By contrast a much earlier Productivity Commission report on regulatory burdens listed 'animal welfare' as a major concern for farmers and the like. Farming groups are now openly attacking RSPCA Australia, claiming it is biased and adopting an extreme view in its policies and positions (for example advocating a ban on live export). Recently, RSPCA Australia has publicly criticised the process for development of animal welfare Standards and Guidelines, saying that those running this process (which is the private organisation, Animal Health Australia) are seeking to selectively refer to animal welfare science which favours the position of the farming lobby. The New South Wales Farmers Association has sought to restrict the inspectorial powers of RSPCA (NSW), accusing it of 'moving to the dark side'.[281] In Western Australia right wing members of the Upper House initiated a lengthy investigation into RSPCA (WA) which similarly sought to undermine the position of the organisation. The Victorian parliament has conducted an investigation into RSPCA (Victoria) and has recently sought to restrict the involvement of that organisation in campaigning on issues such as live export. In this regard, it is likely the farming lobby will prevail.

### The core statutes

The division of responsibility between states and the Commonwealth is based on the absence of a specific 'head of power' in the Australian *Constitution* relating to animal welfare. Thus the states, with their power to legislate for 'order and good governance', can legislate in the area of animal welfare.

As a result, the majority of animal welfare law is concentrated in statutes of the States and Territories. There are some areas, such as live export and slaughter of animals for production of meat for export, which are the preserve of the Commonwealth, laws being passed under the 'trade and commerce' and 'external affairs' heads of power in the Australian *Constitution*.[282] Here the references to animal welfare are incidental to the expressed powers.[283] There are some other areas, such as biosecurity and treatment of wildlife, where there is overlap between the Commonwealth and states and territories jurisdictions.

I agree completely with the view that '...the animal welfare acts are a patchwork of conflicting and confusing definitions'.[284] A defining feature of the main animal welfare statutes is their lack of consistency. This situation is likely to continue for the foreseeable future, given the Commonwealth has walked away from its coordinating role.

---

[281] see Goodfellow (2015).
[282] s51(i); s51(xxix).
[283] s51(xxxix).
[284] Walker-Munro (2015).

Lawmakers have lost sight of the need to be simple and direct. In this regard, John Webster points to the second definition of cruelty in the UK *Protection of Animals Act 1911*, as being simple and direct: it is an offence 'to cause unnecessary suffering by doing, or omitting to do any act'; he also notes the inclusion of a duty of care in the UK *Animal Welfare Act 2006*, which has the effect of imposing a duty not only to avoid conditions leading to suffering, but also to do things which promote positive welfare outcomes.[285] This is, perhaps, as much as is needed. Everything else is a gloss. The only detail needed in the law is to set out what is 'unnecessary'. In Australia at present this is in effect dictated by industry, such that 'usual farming practices' are exempted from the operation of the law (see below).

The laws are all parts of the criminal law, so proof of an offence must reach the criminal standard of 'beyond reasonable doubt'. This is a very high bar to set, which perhaps explains why many regulatory authorities turn to prosecution as the last resort.

All of the modern anti-cruelty and animal welfare statutes in Australia make it an offence to be cruel to *an animal*, or to neglect the welfare of *an animal*; that is, the focus is on the individual. The statutes also impose a range of positive duties on relevant persons, such as the duty to make sure animals are properly fed.

### Qualifiers and defences

The core cruelty and welfare provisions are in essence qualified. 'Cruelty' at law is not cruelty *per se*, but cruelty which is 'unreasonable' and 'unnecessary'. And cruelty can be found to be reasonable or necessary for the most trivial of reasons. These sorts of terms came into the English law in 1849, adopting the view expressed by pioneers like Richard Martin.[286] The leading case on this issue is *Ford v Wiley*.[287] In that case, Lord Coleridge CJ said 'the mere infliction of pain, even if

---

[285] Webster (2005).
[286] Radford (2001), 199.
[287] (1889) 23 QBD 203.

extreme pain, is manifestly not by itself sufficient' to amount to cruelty. Suffering can be inflicted only if it is 'necessary'.

In Australia, the only recent case which analyses the meaning of these words in animal cruelty legislation is the *Al Kuwait* case, dealt with by the Perth Magistrates Court in Western Australia.[288] In that case, Crawford M referred to *Ford v Wiley*, citing Coleridge CJ's comment, regarding 'necessary', that

> *'we may perhaps approach a definition from the negative. There is no necessity and it is not necessary to sell beasts for 40s more than could otherwise be obtained for them; nor to pack away a few more beasts in a farm yard, or a railway truck, than could otherwise be packed; nor to prevent a rare and occasional accident from one unruly or mischievous beast injuring others. These things may be convenient or profitable to the owners of cattle, but they cannot with any show of reason be called necessary. That without which an animal cannot attain its full development or be fitted for its ordinary use may fairly come within the term 'necessary' and if it is something to be done to the animal it may fairly and properly be done.'*

She noted that the principle emerging from the judgments in *Ford v Wiley* was that necessity requires proportion between the object and the means. I cite this lower court case for the reason that no other reported Australian cruelty case even mentions *Ford v Wiley* in this context. But I think it will still be regarded as good law in Australia.

When one looks in detail at what was said in *Ford v Wiley*, a clear picture emerges, as illustrated by the following passages:

From Coleridge CJ:

---

[288] *Department of Local Government & Regional Development v Emanuel Exports Pty Ltd & Ors* (unreported) Magistrates Court of Western Australia FR9975-7/05;FR10225-7/05, Crawford M.

*'...as to necessity, it is found in the case that for twenty years the practice of dishorning has been entirely disused throughout England and Wales. It has not been thought necessary in all that time to perform it on any of the millions of cattle which during that time the farmers of England of all sorts have reared...It is incredible to me, at least, that an operation for many years discontinued in England and Wales, and [the cited exception]...in Scotland also, should suddenly have become 'necessary' so as to except it, if it be cruel, from the mischiefs against which the statute is directed.'*

Relevant evidence cited was that of a Professor from the Royal (Dick) Veterinary College at Edinburgh, who noted that the 'English National Congress of Veterinary Surgeons' had passed resolutions condemnatory of cattle dishorning. There was further evidence from other Professors of Veterinary Surgery condemning the practice. Coming from the other side, the farmers sought to establish that, even though the operation caused pain, it was possible to get dehorned animals closer together in a yard, and 'butchers pay more' for 'polled than for horned beasts'. Lord Coleridge's response to that was as set out in the *Al Kuwait* case above.

From Hawkins J:

*'It would be unreasonable to claim for domestic animals designed for man's use absolute immunity from all suffering at the hand of man; and it would not be contended by the strongest advocates of the cause of humanity that pain to some extent may not be reasonably inflicted with a view to save an animal's life, to cure it from sickness or injury, or to fit it to fulfil the part for which by common consent it is designed. In each case, however, the beneficial or useful end sought to be attained must be reasonably proportionate to the extent of the suffering caused, and in no case can substantial suffering be inflicted, unless necessity for its infliction can reasonably be said to exist. To save the life of an animal, to restore it to health when suffering from painful disorder, violent measures, causing much misery to it, may oftentimes be matter of necessity; a wounded*

*or diseased limb, or an injured eye, may require surgical treatment inseparable from pain; these are illustrations of cases in which the pain caused is for the direct benefit of the animal itself...*

*But a striking body of evidence that such an operation is unnecessary and unreasonable is to be found in the fact that throughout vast districts, both in England and Scotland, thousands upon thousands of horned cattle are to be seen, many herding together peacefully enough, grazing in the same fields, confined in the same yards, feeding, thriving and fattening together, and packed together in railway trucks for transportation to market.'*

The conclusion from all of this is that, while cruelty, to be 'necessary' and 'reasonable', must be proportionate to the object, to some extent it can be seen that the judgment as to what was proportionate to an object was based on whether or not the practice was usual. Thus, if a sufficient majority of farmers carried out a particular practice, which of itself was cruel, then it could be regarded as necessary and reasonable.

Although there is no reported Australian case concerning the interpretation of the words 'unnecessary' or 'unreasonable', the commentary by Mike Radford on the position in the UK is invaluable. He particularly points to the modern decision regarding veal crates, *Roberts v Ruggiero*, where Stephen Brown LJ said 'the magistrates did not find that suffering was caused to any of the calves in this instance beyond that which was general in animal husbandry'.[289] It therefore appears that the English courts have interpreted these words in the context of what is usual acceptable practice. Thus, in *Hall v RSPCA*[290] the questions asked by the court included whether the practices the subject of the case would have been carried out by '...a reasonably competent, reasonably humane modern pig farmer...'. As Radford said, if a defendant was able to produce evidence that a significant body of competent and humane pig farmers would find the suffering acceptable, he might be acquitted. So the standards applied to

[289] QBD, 3 April 1985, referred to in Radford (2001).
[290] QBD, 11 November 1993, referred to in Radford (2001).

determine what is reasonable or necessary are the 'prevailing standards within the industry'. This is extremely important, because it means that common farming practices, no matter how cruel, are excused simply because they are commonly used. This is a major problem with the modern law – I have yet to see it even raised in Australia.

In more modern times, the animal use industries have become increasingly nervous about the application of animal cruelty law to the practices they inflict on animals. Consequently, they have for some time sought to render themselves immune from the reach of the animal cruelty law when these practices are employed. Clearly in doing so, they have thereby indirectly acknowledged that the practices are cruel, and that the economic interests driving their use will prevail over animal welfare considerations.[291]

Jed Goodfellow (2015) has set out a useful history of the development of 'defences' in the statutes, whereby certain practices, if carried out in a certain way, do not constitute offences under the acts. Thus practices such as dehorning of cattle, castration, branding, tail docking and so on were exempted by relevant sections of the core acts.

Over the years, an important component of the qualification of what is 'cruel' at law has been the development of animal welfare 'model codes of practice'. Neumann (2005) noted that the development of the relevant Pig Code was initiated by the pork industry because of

> 'concern...over changes to welfare practices and the continued acceptability of sow stalls in the European Union, the United Kingdom and in New Zealand. That imperative has sought to manage change rather than have it imposed on the industry as could foreseeably result from successful lobbying by animal welfare advocacy groups.'

---

[291] Goodfellow (2015).

Neumann (2005) also noted that involvement of industries in Code development was based on documenting existing management practices; industry felt that compliance should be voluntary.

In essence, many (but not all) of the relevant statutes provide for a defence against a prosecution for breach of the law if there has been compliance with the relevant code of practice. However, this position has been undermined in recent years as there is now no centralised system, accountable to a parliament, relating to the codes of practice. For a time this role was filled by the Australian Animal Welfare Strategy (AAWS), but this operation was abandoned in 2013, when the Commonwealth withdrew all funding. This coincided with the disbanding of the Commonwealth Department of Agriculture's Animal Welfare Branch.[292]

There has been a concerted move towards substitution of the codes of practice by 'Standards and Guidelines'.[293] The intention was (and probably still is) that each code be replaced by 'Standards and Guidelines' which would be endorsed by all of the states and territories ministers with responsibility for animal welfare. The intention was that the endorsed 'Standards', expressed in mandatory terms, would then be incorporated into the relevant legislation. This would happen either by the words of the 'Standards' being picked up in regulations made under the relevant statutes, or by reference to the 'Standard' in the relevant legislation.

Note, however, that this approach is very different from an approach whereby acceptable practices are set out in codes, such that compliance with the codes can be a defence to prosecution. The current approach comes at the issue from the opposite perspective. Rather than saying what can be done, the Standards say what cannot be done. When the relevant model code of practice ceases to exist, having been supplanted by the 'Standards and Guidelines', there seems to have been no

---

[292] Goodfellow (2015).
[293] See Bloom (2008) regarding the history of this development.

provision made for what happens to the defences available under some of the state and territory legislation. As things stand, it looks as if there will be two tiers of documents; the 'Standards', which will become mandatory through regulations (or some other form of adoption by the relevant law) and outdated codes, which will just sit there and act as defences in those jurisdictions which have defence provisions.

The role of the 'Guidelines' is not clear. It seems they represent aspirations, rather than practices which everyone should adhere to. My view is that because of this they are worthless and pointless.

### *Animal welfare standards*

As already noted, in 2005 Dr Geoff Neumann was commissioned by the then federal Department of Agriculture to review the development processes for the Australian Model Codes of Practice for the Welfare of Animals. One of his key recommendations was that the Codes of Practice should be replaced by mandatory Standards. In a sense, his recommendation was accepted, but in a heavily modified way. For example, he made the logical and sensible suggestion that the first step in the development of a new Standard should be that 'an independent animal welfare science review be carried out'. This has not happened, and in fact the process which has evolved is neither documented, enforceable, or independent.

With the demise of the Australian Animal Welfare Strategy, the private company Animal Health Australia assumed the leadership role in the development of animal welfare Standards. The members of this company are animal use industry organisations including the Australian Chicken Meat Federation, Australian Egg Corporation Limited, Australian Pork Limited, the Cattle Council, as well as agriculture representatives of the various Australian governments. On its face, it seems that the process of devising Standards is set out in the relevant Animal Health Australia 'Business Plan'. For each Standard, a key body is the 'writing group', made up of industry and government representatives, as well as (it is claimed) 'independent science representation' and an 'independent chair'. In recent years, however, neither Animals Australia or RSPCA Australia have participated in the 'writing groups', as their view is that their involvement will have little impact.[294] There is a 'stakeholder reference group' which reviews and provides comment on what is produced by the 'writing group'. The aim is to settle a draft for public consultation. At the same time as this is produced, the writing group produces a Regulatory Impact Statement. Once public consultation is complete, all parties attempt to produce a final draft for endorsement by the relevant ministers. This takes place in an *ad hoc* forum of agriculture ministers: 'AgMin'.[295]

Glenys Oogjes, Executive Director of Animals Australia, has been a participant in and observer of these processes for many years. She notes that the process is highly biased towards serving the interest of the animal use industries. There is no attempt to produce an independent review of the relevant scientific literature. The Regulatory Impact Statements are produced by a firm of economic consultants, and the science which is referenced is selected to favour the industry standpoint. The voice of those interested in animal welfare is in effect drowned out by the overwhelming majority, which are the representatives of industry.[296]

There are echoes of this in the 2017 report of the Productivity Commission, *Regulation of Australian Agriculture*. It said that 'the standard setting process does not adequately value the benefits of animal welfare to the community'. It went on to say that community confidence should be improved by measures including more reliance on rigorous science and evidence of community values for animal welfare, and more independent and robust application of regulatory impact assessment processes. The report goes on to illustrate the complete mess that is the process today. It gives the example of the development

---

[294] Goodfellow (2015).
[295] see Goodfellow (2015); Productivity Commission (2017).
[296] see Caulfield (2017); Productivity Commission (2017).

of the sheep and cattle standards, where WA Farmers claimed that RSPCA WA had approved the standards, while RSPCA WA said the cattle and sheep representatives threatened to withhold funding for the review process until they got what they wanted. The latter is certainly my recollection.

The latest animal welfare standards under review are those for poultry. Perhaps unsurprisingly, the process and outcome of the deliberations over the last few years appear to have been stage-managed to suit industry requirements. For example, the science on layer hen housing quoted in the Regulatory Impact Statement[297] is based on questionable techniques (with the now traditional Australian emphasis on 'stress hormone' measures) and consists of a high number of reviews referencing unpublished work, unpublished reviews, industry reports, and in one notable case, a PhD thesis. This is a travesty.

There are other strong indications of bias towards industry in the process. Documents obtained by Dr Jed Goodfellow of RSPCA Australia from the New South Wales Department of Primary Industries, under freedom of information legislation, have revealed what appears to be serious collusion between that department and industry interests in the conduct of the review.[298] The evidence is that the whole process was 'stage-managed', including holding secret meetings between industry players and department representatives in order to do things including 'to stifle moves to review some of the growing scientific evidence that showed chickens suffered in camped cages'. The secret group made statements including that meetings with animal welfare groups should 'avoid close discussion of statistics'. A senior veterinary officer appeared to advocate removing a statement that chickens should have sufficient space to stand and stretch limbs, simply because this was impossible in a battery cage. In other words, a basic behavioural

---

[297] http://www.animalwelfarestandards.net.au/poultry/poultry-public-consultation/.
[298] see www.abc.net.au/news/2017-12-21/egg-farmers-accused-of-colluding-with-nsw-government/9229242

freedom could not be considered, simply because if it was, it would preclude the continued use of battery cages. In response to what seems to be a completely failed and corrupt process, the Victorian government has commissioned its own review into the welfare of poultry. That review was carried out by the experts at Bristol University, led by Professor Christine Nicol.[299] The Western Australian Minister for Agriculture, Alannah MacTiernan, has also expressed disquiet about what seems to be a very unsatisfactory process. This disturbing exercise confirms what many animal welfare advocates have suspected for decades, which is that the government authorities involved in setting animal welfare standards view their role as being to act in the industry's best interests; the interests of animals comes a very poor second. This is nothing more than corruption. Interestingly, Animals Australia has said in this context that it has referred the matter to the New South Wales Independent Commission Against Corruption.[300]

The conclusion is that the current Standards creation process is broken. The recent Productivity Commission report highlights several examples. For instance, those running the process for development of standards for slaughter have seemingly ruled that non-stun (ie religious) slaughter would not be a subject for discussion.[301] This is outrageous. As the Commission said, there is no legitimate reason for this issue to be excluded from the standards development process. Moreover, the report expressly refers to concerns about industry dominance in setting standards. With the revelations concerning the poultry standards, for the first time there is what looks very like hard evidence of the inadequacy of this system.

### Enforcement
After its foundation in the early 1800s, the organisation which became the (English) RSPCA fairly rapidly evolved into an entity which

---

[299] Nicol et al. (2017).
[300] Glenys Oogjes, Executive Director Animals Australia 21 December 2017.
[301] Productivity Commission (2017).

energetically pursued cruelty prosecutions. Indeed the original RSPCA inspectors were described as 'constables'.[302]

The model for enforcement of animal cruelty law in Australia, unsurprisingly, had the English RSPCA as its basis. To the public, the RSPCA has the primary role in detecting breaches of the anti-cruelty and animal welfare statues, and is recognised as being responsible for prosecuting those breaches. All RSPCAs are charities, although many receive some funding from the states governments for their inspectorate function. Even so, this funding is well below the level required to do a proper job. I have always maintained that it is completely inappropriate for a charitable body to be involved in the enforcement of part of the criminal law.[303] Also, as Elizabeth Ellis has pointed out, this outsourcing of animal welfare law enforcement to a charity sends the message that this matter is 'less deserving of attention than other areas of public policy'.[304]

RSPCAs have several conflicts of interest. The first is that in taking an 'advocacy' position on animal welfare issues (primarily through their association with the federal body, RSPCA Australia), there is a perception that they cannot act without bias in carrying out investigation and prosecutorial duties.[305] This perceived conflict has been used as a stick which can be employed to beat RSPCAs by those who want to do so. Another point which is rarely mentioned is that RSPCAs themselves arguably would not want to give up the investigation and prosecution sides of their activities, if only because it creates a good impression with the public, which in turn may be influenced to donate more. But that is just an opinion.

Because RSPCAs receive government funding for their inspectorate functions, those in government who dislike the way they operate can

---

[302] Harrison (1973),
[303] Caulfield (2009).
[304] Ellis (2012).
[305] Comrie (2016)

use the government funding to influence how the RSPCA behaves. For example, in Western Australia (where the RSPCA receives $500,000 per annum from the government) an Upper House MP for the Shooters and Fishers Party managed to instigate a parliamentary inquiry into the operation of the RSPCA (WA).[306] Arguably, the inquiry was instigated because those having farming interests were concerned that the RSPCA was being 'taken over' by 'radical animal liberationists' and the organisation was 'anti-farming'. Much of this seems to have been stimulated by RSPCA (WA)'s support for a ban on live export.[307] The gist of its recommendations was that responsibility for prosecution be centred in the WA Agriculture Department. It would probably not be outlandish to suggest this is what the instigators of the inquiry wanted because they would regard the Agriculture Department as being inclined to support animal users in a way RSPCA (WA) would not. As this inquiry was conducted while a Coalition government was in power, and there is now a Labor government in WA, it appears moot that any of the inquiries' recommendations will be implemented. Nevertheless, some telling points emerged from this inquiry, including the admission by the Agriculture Department CEO that his department had no 'overarching and comprehensive strategic plan and policy for animal welfare in Western Australia'.[308]

At the present time, administration, and to some extent enforcement of anti-cruelty and animal welfare laws in Australia is the responsibility (usually) of the state or territory department dealing with agriculture, set out in Table 1.

---

[306] Select committee into the operations of the Royal Society for the Prevention of Cruelty to Animals Western Australia (Inc) (2016).

[307] See the minority report by Lynn MacLaren MLC and Dr Sally Talbot MLC.

[308] Minority Report para 36: Select committee into the operations of the Royal Society for the Prevention of Cruelty to Animals Western Australia (Inc) (2016).

*Table 1*         Departments responsible for administration of animal
                  cruelty prevention and welfare laws

| Jurisdiction | Department |
|---|---|
| Queensland | Department of Agriculture, Fisheries and Forestry |
| New South Wales | Department of Primary Industries |
| Australian Capital Territory | Territory and Municipal Services |
| Victoria | Department of Economic Development, Jobs, Transport and Resources |
| Tasmania | Department of Primary Industries, Water and Environment |
| South Australia | Department of Environment, Water and Natural Resources |
| Western Australia | Department of Primary Industries and Regional Development |
| Northern Territory | Department of Primary Industry and Fisheries |

In many states, the responsible department has agreed a Memorandum of Understanding with the relevant RSPCA which has the effect of excluding that organisation from enforcement of the law where farmed animals are involved. This is the case in Queensland, Victoria and Western Australia.[309] RSPCA inspectors in New South Wales must seek advice from the relevant department before charging a person with an offence in relation to a 'stock animal'.[310]

Goodfellow (2015), in his study of regulators of animal welfare in agriculture departments, found that the regulatory style was focused on 'compliance' rather than 'deterrence'. There was a considerable emphasis on 'co-regulation'; in other words, inspection responsibilities

---

[309] see Productivity Commission (2017).
[310] section 8(4) *Prevention of Cruelty to Animals Act 1979*.

could be left to industry quality assurance programmes. Victoria is the only state where the legislation expressly contemplates co-regulation. The *Livestock Management Act 2010* (Vic) allows the recognition of an industry quality assurance programme, which can then be authorised in an approved compliance arrangement. Where this happens, the persons who are the subject of the quality assurance programme do not have to comply with the requirement in section 7 of that Act to conduct a systematic risk assessment. They are also deemed to comply with the requirements in the Act and thereby will not be subject to inspections; the government role is to review the reports of third party auditors.

It ought to be obvious that the only way to properly enforce animal welfare law, particularly where animals are used commercially, is for those charged with enforcing the law to be able to carry out random inspections of premises where animals are kept. This is not the case in several major jurisdictions. In Western Australia, an inspector may only enter a place to check on animal welfare (where there is no evidence of emergency, and application has not been made for a warrant) if at least 24 hours notice has been given – and the owner or occupier does not object. In the event there is an objection, a lengthy review process is triggered. Hardly conducive to ensuring animal welfare is a priority. In Queensland there is no provision for random inspections. In Victoria a 'specialist inspector' (appointed by the Minister) may in effect conduct random inspections. It is not clear why this is not automatically a power granted to all animal welfare inspectors.

In Australia and in other parts of the world, animal protection groups dissatisfied with what they see as the failure of laws to adequately protect animals, have trespassed on commercial enterprises which use animals in order to expose cruel practices. This usually involves intensive animal operations, such as intensive piggeries or chicken operations which use battery cages. The public reaction to media reports of such practices has inevitably been one of horror. Even though the evidence has been obtained illegally, and can therefore be excluded from legal proceedings at the discretion of the relevant judicial officer, on several recent occasions that discretion has been exercised to allow the evidence in. In many instances that evidence has resulted in criminal convictions. The most recent such examples have included examples of using live animals to encourage greyhounds to chase a lure (live baiting).

The failure of the present enforcement system is illustrated by the fact that the bulk of evidence showing high levels of cruelty and non-compliance with the law in recent years has come from the activities of non-government organisations, or individuals, albeit engaging in trespass.[311] It could almost be said that the public expects there to be monitoring by non-government organisations such as Animals Australia and Animal Liberation, to the extent that this is regarded as the acceptable norm. In responding to these revelations, both industry and governments refuse to accept that there is a systemic problem. Indeed, such exposure has led to a backlash from the animal use industries. A typical reaction is for farmers to say that the cruelty which has been exposed is atypical, or that the animal protection groups did not tell the enforcement authorities sufficiently soon after they obtained the evidence, because they wanted to make a splash with the media. There is no doubt that the existing criminal law relating to trespass and damage is adequate to deal with illegal entry onto farming properties, and in many jurisdictions there are laws which prohibit the covert installation of surveillance devices. Indeed, Chris Delforce and Dori Kiss were recently charged under the relevant Act in New South Wales, after a warrant to search their homes had been executed. Fortunately for them, the case failed on a technicality. However, not content with the existing law, some politicians whose interests align with the animal use industries have responded to the upset of their audiences by proposing laws which impose draconian penalties for these sorts of surveillance activities. Such legislation is referred to as 'ag-gag'. This has been particularly prevalent in the United States.

---

[311] see, for example, the incidents referred to by Ellis (2012).

So far as the US is concerned, several polls have showed that a majority of the public are opposed to ag-gag laws. Even in the animal use industry, some of those surveyed have expressed the view that such laws may create the impression that the industry has something to hide. Of course the latter may well be true. Robbins et al. (2016) carried out an interesting survey which showed that, when learning of ag-gag legislation, the overwhelming response of those informed was to express reduced trust in farmers. This was so regardless of whether the subjects ate meat or not. Moreover, the participants in the survey on learning about ag-gag laws expressed increased support for better animal welfare laws.

The bottom line on enforcement of the law, particularly as it relates to farm animals, is that it is inadequate. There should be a root and branch review of this issue across the country, which should have as a major aim the recruitment of farmers and animal users to a culture of observance and compliance. There must be powers for random inspections, which should be carried out and reported routinely. This can only happen when there is a national independent body with responsibility for animal welfare.

### Strategic litigation

Surveys say there is a substantial majority in Australia who believe that existing laws purporting to protect animals are inadequate.[312] This misses the point. It is attitudes which are inadequate. Animal welfare is one of those issues that everybody says they are concerned about, but which never quite makes it onto the mainstream political agenda. That said, in my view, 'the law' is almost inevitably not the answer to the problems of animals in Australia. I have often heard it said that one needs to have 'strategic litigation' in order to improve things. A decade ago I might have agreed. But not now. Dawn Lowe, Naomi Sharp[313] and I started such a test case in the Federal Court, relating to the failure of

---

[312] Faunalytics Animal Tracker Australia – Baseline Report 2014.
[313] Of the New South Wales Bar; elected Senior Counsel in October 2017.

the Department of Agriculture to properly enforce the law relating to live export.[314] Apart from Animals' Angels being granted standing on appeal (of which, more below),[315] the case failed in every respect. It probably cost Animals' Angels something like $150,000 altogether. 'Strategic litigation' is a waste of time because animal laws in Australia are in the main written to be immune from challenge by interest groups. To be blunt, people prefer to talk about an attractive-sounding idea, but don't want to be faced with the ugly reality. Fortunately for me, I am not alone in this view. Eminent animal lawyer Jonathon Lovvorn (2006) talked about the daydream: *'if we simply find the right legal and scientific arguments, with the right animals, on the right day, with the right judge, we will have an epic courtroom struggle in which the inalienable legal rights of animals will be declared once and for all'*.

---

[314] *Animals' Angels eV v Secretary, Department of Agriculture* [2014] FCA 398.
[315] *Animals' Angels eV v Secretary, Department of Agriculture* [2014] FCAFC 173. With the generous assistance of Dr JK Kirk SC.

# Chapter 6    Eating Meat (and other animal use)

The current position adopted by most economic commentators and analysts is that economic growth is essential. Growth is inevitably associated with increased population, increased wealth (for some) and increased consumption and demand for animal food products. Raworth (2017) argues persuasively that this model is neither necessary nor desirable. There is absolutely no sign that anyone is taking any notice of that point of view. This mad self-destructive scheme will ultimately surely destroy the human species and a lot more other species as well. In the meantime, we will continue subjecting animals to cruelty on a grand and growing scale.

## Farming animals

In considering the raising and killing of animals for food and other materials, we are at the nub of the animal welfare problem. Farming animals is inevitably associated with cruelty. Peter Singer quotes at length from the UK *McLibel* trial to illustrate this, and refers to testimony from the chief executive of one of McDonald's major suppliers, who in response to the question from Helen Steel (one of the defendants, representing herself) whether it was true 'as the result of the meat industry, the suffering of animals is inevitable', said 'the answer must be yes'.[316] There is a clear conflict between maintenance of animal welfare and the productivity demands of the animal farming industry.[317]

Humans have been farming animals for a very long time. For example, it is known that sheep were domesticated some 11,000 years ago; however 'farming' animals as such probably started about 2,500 to

---

[316] Singer (2000), referring to *McDonald's Corporation and McDonald's Restaurants Limited v Steel and Morris* QBD 19 June 1997. The action was brought by McDonald's against two activists who had made statements in literature about the way animals used in the supply of McDonald's products were raised.
[317] Goodfellow (2015).

3,500 BCE, as evidenced by Egyptian depictions of cattle farming.[318] The basic techniques of farming have therefore been practised for thousands of years. Farmed animals are deprived of their freedom. Where they are grown to be killed and eaten, the females are made pregnant as frequently as possible. Their offspring are taken away from them and grown until they are big enough to be killed and yield profitable amounts of meat. The same applies where animals (usually cattle) are farmed in order to produce milk. Cows have to be made pregnant and give birth in order to lactate as much as possible. In the case of a milk-producing enterprise, the male cattle are in essence by-products, and are got rid of (ie killed at a slaughterhouse) as soon as possible – these are the 'bobby calves'. A similar thing happens where chickens are kept to produce eggs. The male chicks are unwanted, and are destroyed as soon as possible.

Another aspect of the use of animals in farming is selective breeding. Humans using animals have for centuries, if not millenia, employed the technique of selective breeding to better suit the animals to human requirements. This has resulted in several problems for the animals concerned. For example, pigs nowadays are so huge their legs just cannot support their weight. Dairy cattle produce so much milk that they are probably in serious discomfort until they are milked.

The numbers of animals involved are substantial. Far and away the most common food animal is the chicken, used for egg production and meat. There are nearly 26 million egg-laying chickens in Australia, producing about 435 million dozen eggs each year.[319] About 630 million chickens were slaughtered for meat in the year 2015-16.[320] There are roughly 23 million beef cattle, 1.7 million dairy cattle, 2.2 million pigs and 70 million

---

[318] Goodfellow (2015).

[319] Australian Egg Corporation Limited *Australian egg industry overview – December 2015*.

[320] Australian Chicken Meat Federation *Industry Facts and Figures* www.chicken.org.au.

sheep.[321] It is difficult to say how many fish and other sea creatures are killed and consumed each year, but the total quantity in 2014-15 was about 240,000 tonnes.[322]

As one would expect, the increase in meat chicken numbers is reflected in the increase in chicken consumption, which now averages about 46kg per person per year. This compares to 28kg for beef, 11kg for lamb and mutton, and 28kg for pig meat. Forty years ago, chicken consumption was less than a third of what it is today.[323]

Although it is generally thought that animal welfare problems are particularly acute where animals are housed in confined spaces, nevertheless extensive farming can be associated with poor animal welfare. In 2017 for the first time reports appeared of cattle deaths in New South Wales during an unprecedented heatwave. It does not seem unreasonable to suggest such events will become more common with global warming. This will be particularly so where animals are farmed almost in the wild, as is the case with cattle and sheep on huge stations in northern Western Australia and the Northern Territory. It is hard to know what the problems are with those animals, as not only are they hardly seen from one year to the next, but also breeding is uncontrolled, so the actual numbers involved are unknown.

When information is obtained about non-intensive farming practices that go on out of sight, it is rarely edifying. In 2016, People for the Ethical Treatment of Animals (PETA) gathered footage of sheep being shorn in typical Australian sheep shearing sheds. The footage showed sheep being killed, punched and kicked.[324] This is of course an example of practices which occur out of the public gaze and which have probably

---

[321] ABARES (2015).
[322] ABARES (2015).
[323] ABARES (2015).
[324] investigations.peta.org/australia-us-wool/.

been going on for many years. It is something of a relief that practices many of us suspected were occurring have at last been exposed.[325]

Growing animals to provide meat for food is very inefficient. The highest level of efficiency, where intensive systems are used, does not even manage to approach the 20% level. Unfortunately, as the demand for meat as a food grows with growing populations and growing average wealth, so there will be an increased demand for 'sustainable' meat production. This will necessarily involve a shift to intensification, as extensive systems are grossly inefficient so far as land use and feed conversion efficiency is concerned.[326]

Surgical mutilation of animals without pain relief is part of everyday farming life. While it is particularly associated with intensive farming, nevertheless, male cattle and sheep are routinely castrated using rubber bands around the testicles, lambs undergo mulesing and cattle have horn buds and horns removed. All of these procedures are intensely painful, and are carried out solely for the benefit of the farmer. The Brambell Report in 1965 condemned surgical mutilations of animals and said they should be carried out with pain relief. This has not been widely adopted in Australia.

Farmers and farmers' organisations constantly claim that they care for their animals, and have animal welfare as a high priority. These statements must be looked at in context. Farmers are in farming to make money. The animals they grow to kill for food or exploit for other products are commodities used in their money-making endeavours. Survey data has shown that farmers focus on welfare issues relating to physical condition and productivity, whereas the public in general is far more concerned with issues like the ability to express natural

---

[325] 'Sheep shearers fined up to $3,000 and disqualified from handling sheep after animal cruelty case in Horsham' ABC Rural, 31 March 2017; www.abc.net.au/news/2017-03-31.sheep-shearer-sentenced-animal-cruelty-horsham/8404874.
[326] Webster (1994).

behaviours and space to move freely. Farmers in general think their animals' welfare was good, while consumers think welfare is not so good.[327] It may well be that some farmers do have a relationship with their animals, in which case they must be very conflicted about the animals' ultimate destiny. The reality surely must be that farmers have to harden their hearts, and that any concern for animal welfare is concern only for those aspects of an animal's wellbeing which when catered for, result in a financial return.

As Don Watson says in his magnificent account of farming life in the Australian bush: *'Farmers...live with the apparently loveless conception of cows, sheep and pigs, and with the death of them...To be a farmer, first let the iron into your soul...'.*[328] Regarding the conflict between caring for the animals and dealing with them as products to be exploited, he comments that *'the business involved...ingeniously polite denial of the brutal reality of our enterprise'.*

Studies show that farmers with lower levels of empathy are those whose animals have the lowest levels of indicators of good welfare. [329] That is surely hardly surprising.

This is, of course, an acknowledgment of the truth. Using animals in farming is a dirty business. But farmers don't want to openly admit that. Ralph Acampora has noted that 'one of the key features of oppressive societies is that they do not acknowledge themselves as oppressive'.[330] Farmers can, I suggest, be regarded as part of such an oppressive society.

Parbery and Wilkinson (2012) carried out a survey in Victoria seeking to identify views on how agriculture should contribute to society. When asked what made a good farmer, only 16% of respondents mentioned

---

[327] Cornish et al. (2016).
[328] Watson (2014).
[329] Westbury et al. (2011).
[330] Acampora (2016).

caring about animal welfare. But when asked how important treating animals humanely was, the mean rating (out of 10) was 8.7. When asked how farmers were succeeding in this regard, the mean rating was 6.8. The conclusion was, therefore, that people wanted to see good animal welfare, but farmers were not succeeding in meeting that expectation. Twenty six percent of people said they had taken some action in relation to farmed animal welfare – the majority said they had changed their shopping habits. Very importantly, the authors found little evidence that those who had taken action were urban, as opposed to rural inhabitants.

In considering farmed animals one must not forget the growth of 'aquaculture' in Australia. This is basically factory farming of fish. The animals are kept in enclosures and fed highly concentrated food. In Australia, the major industry involves growing salmon, and it is primarily located in Tasmania. In 2012-13 that segment alone was worth nearly half a billion dollars. [331] There are significant questions regarding the sustainability of the practices involved in industrial aquaculture, and there must inevitably be issues relating to pollution, environmental damage, and animal welfare.[332] There are predictions that the planet will eventually source all its fish from fish farming, as wild sea fish will all but disappear.[333]

**Farming and regulation of animal welfare**
The regulation of the use of animals in farming is particularly difficult. Farmers energetically maintain that they know what is good for their animals and because they want their animals to be productive, then that necessarily means the animals' welfare is good. This is, of course, untrue. The primary conflict for a farmer is that she or he is primarily motivated by commercial considerations, that is, making a profit. The welfare of the animals concerned is therefore secondary. Combine this

---

[331] ABARES (2014) Australian fisheries and aquaculture statistics 2013.

[332] Broom and Fraser (2007); Vidal, J 'Salmon farming in crisis: 'we are seeing a chemical arms race in the seas''. *The Guardian* 1 April 2017.

[333] see Compassion in World Farming at www.ciwf.org.uk/farm-animals/fish/.

with the high regard the public has for farmers (which some would say is completely unjustified) and this makes for a very difficult situation for regulators.

Chapter 5 sets out the 'qualifiers and defences' in the law, most of which allow farmers to carry out 'usual husbandry practices'. It is my belief that even in jurisdictions where it is not spelled out, the qualifier that cruelty must be 'unreasonable and unnecessary' to breach the law will serve to protect farmers who can say that what they are doing is no more than applying usual practice.

But there is another important point, which is whether the cruelty which is inflicted by virtue of raising animals which ultimately are to be eaten amounts to something which is 'necessary'. In this case, the 'necessity' relates to whether a person needs to feed on parts of an animal. This is addressed below.

The general animal cruelty / welfare law protects each individual animal. An act of cruelty against one animal, or failure to look after one animal, is an offence. Understandably, farmers don't like this idea and claim that animal welfare legislation is 'outdated in terms of modern farming practices, because it focuses mainly on the individual animal, versus caring for the herd...'.[334] This is a pernicious and dangerous view and should be energetically rejected.

There is much more acceptance that a substantial number of consumers are prepared to pay more for better animal welfare. This, however, is never going to offer a complete solution. The view of the Productivity Commission is that where consumers are not prepared to pay, there should be a minimum level of welfare, regarded as a public good, which should be achieved by government intervention. Thus, the role of government should, they say, be confined to addressing instances where farm animal welfare and profitability are not complementary. The challenge for government is determining the level of farm animal

---

[334] Pearson et al. (2007).

welfare that provides the highest net benefits to the community as a whole.[335]

There is a very good argument for retailers (where possible) imposing animal welfare standards on farmers. This has happened with Coles and Woolworths in Australia.[336] Clearly, such standards can be very effective, as the penalty for breach is felt by the farmer's wallet.[337]

The globalisation of many commodity markets has the potential to greatly influence the welfare of farmed animals in Australia. Although I am always cynical of attempts by the animal users to defend their profits, I think it is entirely reasonable to consider that if one improves animal welfare of farmed animals in Australia, there is the risk that the market will negate any improvements simply because cheaper products can be imported from less animal welfare-friendly jurisdictions.[338] The classical example is import of processed meats (especially pork-based products) from countries which still use extreme confinement, such as sow stalls.[339] It may be that Australia can exclude products from countries which it regards as having unacceptable animal welfare practices, as the World Trade Organization recently upheld a ban on such a basis by the European Union on the import of all seal products.[340] This decision was based on an interpretation of Article XX of the General Agreement on Tariffs and Trade, or GATT, which Australia is bound by.[341] That article enables the imposition of trade barriers on criteria including being 'necessary to protect human, animal or plant life or health'. The decision has been criticised as adopting an 'unduly empiricist definition of public morals and legitimate objectives'.[342]

---

[335] (2017) *Regulation of Australian Agriculture*.
[336] See Caulfield (2017).
[337] Broom (2009).
[338] Grethe (2007).
[339] See Kelch (2016) for a general discussion.
[340] Sellheim (2016).
[341] See Australian Treaty Series 1995 No 8 (Marrakesh Agreement establishing the World Trade Organization).
[342] Herwig (2016).

Regardless, it may open the door for excluding welfare-unfriendly products.

It is clear that Australia is well behind many other developed countries in terms of initiatives to improve the lives of farmed animals. The European Union has removed battery cages for egg-laying chickens and has greatly reduced the use of sow stalls. Similar changes have occurred in New Zealand and in several states of the United States. The Canadian government has moved to get rid of sow stalls.[343]

The animal use industries in Australia essentially dictate the way their practices are regulated. They have control over development of legislation and more or less control research funding. As Goodfellow (2015) puts it, 'animal protection representatives and the broader community are by no means equal participants in the process and their views are not given the same weight as those of the livestock industries'.

Another important point I have already mentioned is that farmers in the main will, I think, engage in a form of civil disobedience if they don't like the 'city folk' trying to regulate them. Jed Goodfellow (2015) thinks the same, based on studies assessing compliance by farmers with environmental controls. As he rightly points out, this tends to create a high risk of non-compliance with animal welfare laws.

In view of all of this, the conclusion has to be that legal regulation of animal use in agriculture must perforce be designed to accommodate and respond to its targets – that is, the farmers. There must be an approach based on education, dialogue and persuasion, rather than coercion. In any case, politicians will not try and coerce farmers because all major political parties are unwilling to provoke a backlash from the powerful farming lobby.

---

[343] See references in Goodfellow (2015).

If one accepts that use of animals in agriculture must be regulated by a non-confrontational approach, then it is inevitable that farming industry representatives will want to base that regulation on quality assurance programmes, that is, self-regulation plus auditing. The corollary of that is, for such a system to be effective, compliance must be regularly monitored. This can only be achieved through unannounced independent inspections and audits at all part of the chains involving animals. So this would include on farms, transport vehicles, markets and saleyards, abattoirs and so on.[344]

The Productivity Commission 2017 report on *Regulation of Australian Agriculture* notes that consumer confidence in regulation of the farm sector use of animals is low, and says that state and territory governments should be more transparent about monitoring and enforcement activities. Industry quality assurance schemes should be part of the picture. I live in hope that a sufficient number of politicians will take this on board and have the courage to do something about it.

### Intensive animal farming ('factory farming')

After the Second World War significant parts of the animal use industries moved to the use of close confinement of animals.[345] In the UK, cutting subsidies in the 1950s put pressure on farmers to increase productivity in order to maintain profit margins. This drove the development and adoption of intensive farming.[346] Most notably, chickens were housed in small cages, veal calves were kept in crates and female pigs were confined to 'stalls' or 'crates' during pregnancy and after giving birth. This was factory farming. These systems were designed to suit those who were keeping the animals. It is easier to feed and monitor an animal, and remove its faeces and urine, when the animal never moves out of a cage for the duration of its life. The number of people required to look after the animals is greatly reduced. Feeding is controlled, uses standardised, processed food, and can be

---

[344] See Broom (2009).
[345] Brambell (1965).
[346] Woods (2011).

automated. The animals' environment can be regulated and kept within limits to maximise productivity. Eventually these systems became entrenched in the animal use industry, and were largely justified on the grounds that other systems were less productive. The meat-consuming public benefitted, because the use of these confinement systems meant less space was consumed, so the product was cheaper. According to Webster (2005), animals in intensive systems probably suffer, for example, by virtue of not being able to modify their diets according to their condition. The same can be said about constraints on other behavioural responses, for example related to regulating body temperature. All options are denied, other than what is provided to them. Another inevitable negative consequence of intensification is proper stockmanship and animal husbandry is no longer an option. The sheer number of animals involved and the high stocking densities makes it impossible to provide anything like the proper level of care and supervision.

The development of intensive farming practices occurred in parallel with the selective breeding of strains of animals which exhibited characteristics which would greatly increase productivity.[347] Perhaps the most obvious example is meat chickens, which now exist in two strains (Cobb and Aviagen) which can grow to slaughter weight (about 2kg) in something like 6 weeks. Pigs have also been selected to grow very quickly, with strains like Large White / Landrace crosses exhibiting phenomenal growth rates. The 'success' from the farming perspective of selective breeding of enormously productive strains of chickens and pigs, as opposed to cows and sheep, is reflected in the data on conversion of food input to meat output. It will come as little surprise that the overall efficiency of meat production is highest for meat chickens and pigs.[348] John Webster (2005) has pointed out that the corollary of this is that the breeding generations of pigs and poultry carry an enormous welfare burden. For example, breeding sows end up

---

[347] see Brambell (1965); Webster (2005).
[348] Webster (2005).

an enormous size, almost too large to support their own weight, and certainly very prone to severe lameness. This means that the cull rate of breeding sows is quite high (they only last a couple of years)[349] but this welfare penalty (in terms of the cost of having to replace culled animals) is compensated for by the high efficiency of the whole system.

It is apparent that today most people dislike the idea that farmed animals should be kept in extreme confinement, such as pigs in sow stalls or egg-laying chickens in battery cages.[350] Other issues with intensive farming include the production of lots of animal waste, which if not controlled can create problems with pollution. Control of infectious diseases is a significant issue for the operators of factory farms.

At the present time, global demand for food is increasing as populations grow, and people in general become wealthier. In rapidly-developing countries with an expanding middle class, such as China and India, demand for meat is rising very quickly. Problems with increased competition for land, water, energy and other inputs to food production are apparent and growing. There have been calls to increase efficiency of food production through 'sustainable intensification'. This may seem like a contradiction in terms, but there may be a sensible underlay. Having said that, few of the discussions relating to the core problem (that is, feeding more people who want more food) identify the causative agents, which must include untrammeled population growth.[351] There is also an unwillingness of people to acknowledge that perhaps they do not need so much food, which includes meat.

The sensible underlay of 'sustainable intensification' may include the need to moderate demand for resource-intensive foods, such as meat

---

[349] see Caulfield (2013).
[350] Faunalytics Animal Tracker Australia – Baseline Report 2014.
[351] One of the few warning against this is Sir David Attenborough: http://www.bbc.com/news/magazine-24303537.

and dairy products, as well as reducing food waste.[352] However, the use of the word 'intensification' necessarily rings warning bells, given its association with farming techniques which result in very poor animal welfare. This means that the goals of 'sustainable intensification' must be contingent on acceptable animal welfare standards.[353]

### Pigs

Pigs have been domesticated for about 9,000 years. Although they would initially have been free to roam about, the development of agriculture resulted in them becoming more confined. Selection for faster growing animals occurred as early as the 18th century.[354]

There are about 2.2 million pigs in Australia, of which approximately 270,000 are breeding sows and gilts (young females).

Intensive pig farming started in Australia in the early 1960s.[355] An intensive pig farm operates with different facilities for the different phases of the pig rearing process. Pregnant sows will be kept in sow stalls (also called gestation stalls, or crates), little bigger than their bodies,[356] until they are ready to give birth. They will then be moved to cages called farrowing crates, which are designed to allow access of piglets to the mother for feeding, while preventing the mother from killing or injuring the piglets by rolling on them. Farrowing crates are even smaller than sow stalls.[357] When piglets are weaned, they are then moved to a grower facility (in a shed), where they grow to the point where they are big enough to be killed at the slaughterhouse.[358]

---

[352] Garnett et al. (2013).
[353] Garnett et al. (2013).
[354] D'Eath and Turner (2009).
[355] Senate Select Committee on Animal Welfare (1990) *Intensive Livestock Production*, p177.
[356] 0.6 metres by 2.2 metres.
[357] 0.5 metres by 2.0 metres.
[358] Marchant-Forde (2009a).

One does not need fancy science to work out that both sow stalls and farrowing crates are cruel - they are just too small. The sow stall is 2.2 metres long and the farrowing crate is 2.0 metres long. These dimensions are only big enough to accommodate a full grown sow if its legs poke through to the next stall, and in any case are not big enough to allow the sow to get up and lie down easily.[359]

The Animal Welfare Code for Pigs in effect allowed the continued use of sow stalls to house pregnant pigs for up to six weeks of every pregnancy. I was part of the Tasmanian Animal Welfare Advisory Committee that advised the Minister not to allow this; that recommendation was made on the basis of detailed consideration of relevant animal welfare science, as well as international economics of pig production in free range systems, and what was being done in other jurisdictions. The pig industry's assertion that the decision was made against the advice of scientific experts is untrue.[360] It is notable that just prior to voting to ban sow stalls, the Committee heard evidence from Professor Paul Hemsworth of the Animal Welfare Science Centre in support of keeping them. However, another animal welfare science expert, Professor John Webster, has said 'those nations that still permit the confinement stall have either not yet reviewed the evidence or chosen to discard [it]'.[361] The Productivity Commission has noted this was a case of a State not endorsing a 'national standard' where it considers that standard to be too low.

After years of vigorously asserting that sow stalls were good for pigs (and saying that was proved by science),[362] in 2010 the Australian pig industry representative body (Australian Pork Limited; APL) voted to 'commit to pursuing the voluntary phasing out of the use of gestation stalls by 2017'. This was probably largely in response to the leading supermarket chain Coles' decision to stop sourcing its own brand pork

---

[359] See Caulfield (2013), 20.
[360] see Caulfield (2013); Productivity Commission (2017).
[361] Webster (2015).
[362] see Caulfield (2013), 13.

from producers which used sow stalls. This announcement was tempered by the statement that producers 'recognise the welfare benefits of gestation stalls'; also, it was followed by a definition of 'gestation stall free' which in effect allowed sows to be kept in sow stalls for 12 days and possibly more (5 days after mating and one week before farrowing).[363] I complained to the Australian Consumer and Competition about the claim by APL in promotional material that Australia was becoming 'gestation stall free'. APL subsequently removed all such material from its website.

Rivalea, which is Australia's biggest pork producer, claims it moved to get rid of sow stalls by 2011. Indeed, it says it received an award from Compassion in World Farming in 2011 for this achievement.[364]

The voluntary ban has not worked. APL is now saying that up to 25% of animals are still in stalls; they admit that the only way to get rid of sow stalls is by legislation.[365] It is informative to note that the aggressive defence of sow stalls by APL up to 2010 was unjustified. The figures for productivity before the ban show that the average number of piglets weaned per sow mated (in 2008/09) was 21.1. After the 'ban' was imposed, average productivity increased to 23 piglets weaned per sow mated (in 2011/2012). This latter figure is almost identical to the productivity of the pig industry in the UK, which does not have sow stalls.[366]

---

[363] The detailed history is presented by me in Caulfield (2013): 'Science and Sense', a report I wrote for Voiceless.

[364] see https://www.rivalea.com.au/Portals/20/Rivalea%20Animal%20Welfare%20-%20Oct%202014.pdf

[365] 'Voluntary sow stall phase-out deadline approaches for last 20 per cent' ABC Rural 22 December 2016; www.abc.net.au/news/2016-12-02/voluntary-sow-stall-phase-out-deadline-approaches/8138450.

[366] Compare APL's Australian Pig Annual for those years.

*Chickens*

Egg-laying chickens were first kept in battery cages in the USA in the 1930s.[367] Battery cages appeared in the UK in the 1960s.[368] The advantages to the chicken farmer are obvious. Faeces can easily be disposed of and feeding and watering can be regimented. Egg producers operate an 'all in, all out' system, whereby birds are brought into the laying sheds when they are old enough to lay ('point of lay'). The birds are hatched usually at a separate establishment. Male chickens (which are obviously unwanted) can be detected the day after hatching by virtue of genetic selection which gives them a different feather colour from females. The males are killed, usually by being put alive into a macerator.

Battery cages have mesh floors, sides and roof, and usually contain four or five birds. So-called 'furnished cages' (with a perch, nest box and area for dust bathing) have been introduced in Europe, but are not used in Australia. Egg producers destock entire sheds (which can contain 25,000 birds) at the same time, which can result in serious mistreatment of the birds. Layer hens are typically kept to about 72 weeks of age, and are then slaughtered.

The outdoor stocking density which must apply if eggs are labelled 'free range' has now been defined as an Information Standard under the Consumer Law; this standard will commence on 18 April 2018.[369] This means that for a package containing eggs to carry the label 'free range', the eggs must be laid by hens that have meaningful and regular access to an outdoor range during daylight hours during the laying cycle, are able to roam and forage on the outdoor range, and that the outdoor stocking density must be no more than 1 hen per square metre. There are no definitions applicable to the housing conditions for the hens,

---

[367] Broom and Fraser (2007).
[368] Woods (2011).
[369] *Australian Consumer Law (Free Range Egg Labelling) Information Standard 2017* (Cth).

which means of course that the stocking density in sheds can be very high and that many hens may never leave the shed.

The negative welfare impacts of battery cage housing are many, and are set out in Chapter 4.

Chickens grown for meat production fare little better, in the main. They are usually kept indoors in sheds housing more than 20,000 birds. The chicken meat industry in Australia is vertically integrated. Two companies control nearly all the market, and they operate the system from hatching to slaughter.[370]

## Surgical mutilations

Farmers frequently adopt surgical procedures to alleviate or prevent problems occurring with farmed animals. These procedures are usually done without local anaesthesia or subsequent pain relief.

The examples of surgical mutilation include mulesing of lambs, castration of calves, lambs and pigs, tooth trimming and tail docking of piglets and beak trimming of chickens. Horned cattle are often dehorned, or horn buds of calves are removed with caustic agents or a hot iron.

Tail-docking of piglets may result in the formation of neuromas in the stump. These often result in severe pain. There is evidence that tail biting will decrease with a reduction in stocking density, but this is more effective when combined with the provision of manipulable material such as straw.[371]

### *Mulesing*

The scientific evidence is that mulesing causes considerable pain, which can be alleviated by use of local anaesthetic. The analgesic effect is greatly enhanced if a non-steroidal anti-inflammatory drug is also used.

---

[370] The companies are Inghams Enterprises Pty Ltd and Baiada Poultry Pty Ltd: Goodfellow (2015).
[371] Broom and Fraser (2007).

The Australian Animal Welfare Standards and Guidelines for Sheep have been endorsed by the states and territories primary industry ministers.[372] It is to be expected the standards will soon become part of Australian law. The Standards (s. 7.3) in effect say that sheep younger than 6 months can be mulesed without the use of pain relief. The vast majority of sheep endure mulesing at less than 6 months of age. The Sheep Decision Regulation Impact Statement expressed the view that 'available scientific research suggests that it is possible to achieve pain relief in conjunction with mulesing'. The Statement also said that there are no non-steroidal anti-inflammatory drugs registered for use in sheep in Australia[373]. This is untrue.

The conclusion is that the development process for the Australian Animal Welfare Standards and Guidelines for Sheep, in approving the continued use of mulesing without pain relief, has ignored the scientific evidence which strongly supports the use of local anaesthetic to relieve pain in mulesed sheep. Furthermore, the recent registration of the non-steroidal anti-inflammatory meloxicam for use in sheep indicates that in any case the assessment process is outdated and should be reviewed.

## Why eat meat?[374]

The majority of Australians eat meat. In 2014, a survey found that about 98% of Australians ate meat. However, the same study found that nearly 65% of those surveyed had bought humane or free range products, and 35% had bought meat alternatives.[375] This is consistent with earlier findings by Adrian Franklin (2007a), who noted that only 6% of Australians he surveyed were vegetarians (interestingly 52% thought factory farming was cruel).[376]

---

[372] www.animalwelfarestandards.net.au/files/2016/02/Sheep-Standards-and-Guidelines-Endorsed-Jan-2016-250116.pdf.
[373] www.animalwelfarestandards.net.au/files/2016/01/Final-Sheep-Decision-RIS-July-2014-300714.pdf.
[374] This discussion will also include reference to dairy products and eggs.
[375] Faunalytics Animal Tracker Australia – Baseline Report 2014.
[376] Franklin (2007).

It seems that as people get richer, so the demand for meat increases. People from less rich nations rely far more on vegetable sources of protein. In India, much protein comes from lentils and rice, while in China the sources are rice, and small amounts of meat and soy. However, meat eating is coming under scrutiny in affluent societies due to perceived environmental and health implications of a high level of meat consumption.[377]

## Nutrition and biochemistry[378]

In order to understand why humans can use meat as a food, and whether eating meat is essential, it is first necessary to understand how we work as living organisms, and the functions of each of the components of food sources.

All living things share the same basic cellular structure. A cell is essentially a container which isolates (in a controlled way) its contents from the outside environment, and which contains the ingredients which allow the organism to function. The outside layer of the cell, or membrane, is made up of particular sorts of lipids (fats), which are oriented to make up two layers. The inner and outer faces are the charged (polar) parts of the lipids, while the parts in the centre are the hydrophobic, uncharged parts of the lipid molecules. Embedded in the lipid membrane are proteins, which serve particular functions, such as responding to signals from the outside (such as hormones, or neurotransmitters – in the case of nerves, muscles, glands and so on), or allowing certain charged particles (ions) to pass back and forth in a controlled fashion (ion channels).

Inside the cell, there are other sub-structures ('organelles'), also made of lipid membranes. The largest and most obvious (which can be seen with a good light microscope) is the cell nucleus. This contains the genetic code (in genes, made of DNA, or deoxyribonucleic acid) which

---

[377] Mathijs (2015).
[378] The main references for this section on nutrition are Smolin and Grosvenor (2013) and Brody (1999).

controls the manufacture of the proteins the cell needs, and also is responsible for passing on genetic material to new cells, and to new organisms as part of the reproductive process. Other important organelles are the mitchondria, which literally provide the power for cell function (generating adenosine trisphosphate; ATP – see below), and the endoplasmic reticulum, which is a kind of protein factory, making the proteins the cell needs (from the building blocks of proteins: amino acids), as instructed by the messages carried from the DNA in the nucleus. The messages are another form of nucleic acid: RNA, or ribonucleic acid.

The key distinction between plant cells and animals (and indeed between plants and animals) is that plants can make their own food, using the energy of the sun – this is photosynthesis; animals, however, must obtain their food by consuming other living organisms (or parts of organisms). The human body requires about 45 nutrients in order to survive. These are substances which the human body cannot make itself. A modern western diet will contain unmodified sources of those essential nutrients, but often some of these nutrients will be added during processing of food. For example, vitamin A might be added to milk.

There are six classes of nutrients: carbohydrates, lipids, proteins, water, vitamins and minerals. Water can be ignored for the purposes of this discussion. Carbohydrates, lipids and proteins, while they perform different roles in the cell's structure, can all be metabolised to provide energy. These energy-yielding nutrients must be consumed in significant quantities (kilograms), so are termed *macronutrients*. In contrast, vitamins and minerals are needed in much smaller quantities (thousands or millionths of grams), so are *micronutrients*.

*Macronutrients*

All of the macronutrients are taken into the body in complex forms, which must be broken down in the gut by digestive processes. The breakdown products are then absorbed into the bloodstream and transported to sites where they are required, and where they are absorbed into cells.

- Carbohydrates give the body a readily available source of energy. They are found in sugars (simple carbohydrates, such as those found in fruits) and in starches (complex chain-like carbohydrates, such as are found in vegetables like potatoes). The basic unit of a carbohydrate is the *monosaccharide*. Molecules which contain one or up to six monosaccharides are called *oligosaccharides*. Monosaccharides and oligosaccharides are sugars, such as glucose and fructose. *Polysaccharides* contain more units; examples are starch, cellulose and glycogen. Indigestible carbohydrates (soluble fibres, resistant starch etc.) have important roles in promoting a healthy gut bacterial population, as they represent a food source for these organisms. Their metabolism by the bacteria generates short-chain fatty acids which are a fuel source for cells in the colon, and serve the additional function of acidifying the colon and inhibiting the growth of undesirable bacteria. However, too much fibre can reduce the absorption of some important micronutrients. Fibre has other beneficial effects, including causing stomach distension (making you feel full) and smoothing out the rate of absorption of nutrients.

- Lipids (fats, oils) represent a highly concentrated form of energy, and as we know to our cost, can be used to store energy in the body. Too much fat, is of course, bad news. Not only do you get fat, but you become prone to diseases including atherosclerosis. The commonest forms of lipid are triglycerides, which are made up of three fatty acids (hence *tri*glyceride). The fatty acids can be *saturated* or *unsaturated*. The degree of saturation tells you how much hydrogen there is in the carbon chains of the fatty acid. This distinction is important when considering the negative health effects of lipids. Lipids are found in foods like meat, dairy products and vegetable oils.

• Proteins, made of chains of amino acids (of which there are twenty), have important structural and metabolic roles. Proteins sourced in the diet are broken down to amino acids, which are then absorbed into the bloodstream from the gut. Amino acids broken down from proteins can also provide energy. Examples of proteins are enzymes (which catalyse the chemical reactions underlying metabolic processes) and the proteins forming the contractile apparatus of muscle (myosin, actin). A catalyst is a substance which greatly accelerates the rate of a particular reaction, without itself being consumed. While proteins are required in a growing body (to make new cells and other body components), proteins are also continually turned over in the body, so a source of new protein is essential even in the adult human. Common food sources of protein are meat, fish, eggs, milk, grains and vegetables. Some amino acids can be made by the body; others have to be obtained from food. Of the 20 amino acids commonly found in protein, 9 cannot be made by the body, and so must be obtained from the diet.[379]

*Micronutrients*

• Vitamins are small organic molecules[380] which play key roles in the biochemical machinery of the body. There are 13 known vitamins. Many of them are involved in the molecular

---

[379] Histidine, isoleucine, leucine, lysine, methionine, phenylalanine, threonine, tryptophan, valine.
[380] Organic molecules are made up of atoms such as carbon, oxygen, nitrogen and sometimes atoms like sulphur.

processes by which energy is released from macronutrient molecules. Others have functions in processes like bone growth, sight, blood clotting and oxygen transport.

- Minerals are 'inorganic'. Well known examples are sodium (in salt as sodium chloride) and calcium. Other examples are potassium and magnesium. Sodium and potassium are essential for the mechanisms by which nerves transmit impulses, and also for the mechanisms underlying muscle contraction. Calcium is needed for normal nerve, muscle and gland function. It is also an essential part of bone structure. Iodine is essential for the functioning of the thyroid, and is routinely added to table salt.

Macronutrients can be either broken down to provide energy, used to make structural molecules, or made into energy storage molecules. So far as energy is concerned, adenosine trisphospate (ATP) is the body's energy currency; ATP is the ultimate product of metabolism of the energy-generating macronutrients. The chemical bonds in ATP are very rich in energy, so when ATP is broken down, a lot of energy is released. That energy is used to power processes in cells, such as muscle contraction, or to provide the electrical potentials in nerves which allow signals to be transmitted. Macronutrients can be broken down in the presence of oxygen, generating the waste products carbon dioxide and water. If oxygen is not present (so-called anaerobic metabolism), the only macronutrients which can be broken down to generate ATP are molecules which produce glucose.

## The nutritional value of meat

It is undeniable that meat is a very good source of protein and other nutrients, including fats, and micronutrients such as iodine, iron, zinc (and other minerals), vitamins (especially $B_{12}$) and essential fatty acids including omega-3 long chain polyunsaturated fatty acids. This latter group of nutrients is especially rich in fish, meat from grass-fed animals, poultry and some eggs. But consumption of high levels of animal products, combined with under-consumption of vegetables and fruit, significantly raises levels of cholesterol, producing a significant increase in the risk of heart disease. So although meat is a good source of many important nutrients, eating too much meat is associated with real risks.

It is interesting that when the current Australian dietary guidelines refer to 'meat', they refer to it as 'lean meat', and lump it in the same class as 'poultry, fish, eggs, tofu, nuts, legumes/beans and seeds'. Firstly, 'lean meat' is important because consuming large amounts of animal fat is thought to be the cause of many of the health risks associated with high meat diets. Secondly, the reference to the other foods, including the non-meat sources, acknowledges that humans are not obligate meat eaters. Humans have long intestinal tracts suited to fermentation by bacterial populations. Carnivores, by contrast, have quite short digestive tracts. Humans have short teeth (and no claws); carnivores have long teeth (and claws). The obvious conclusion is that one does not have to eat meat (lean or otherwise) in order to obtain sufficient protein to live healthily. To quote John Webster, *'we do not all 'need' animals to provide us with food. It is relatively easy for a non-lactating adult to thrive on a vegan diet and possible, though more difficult, for a growing child'*.[381] It is not 'necessary' to eat meat, and therefore not 'necessary' to grow animals to eat, and so cruelty inflicted as a result of growing those animals is not 'necessary', and therefore, strictly speaking, is illegal (see Chapter 5). However, there is no chance of a magistrate or judge convicting a farmer on this basis. What this means in practical terms is the legal definition of 'necessary' is quite different from the dictionary definition of 'necessary' ('required to be done', according to my Oxford Concise). The legal meaning of the word is what Humpty Dumpty said to Alice: 'just what I choose it to mean';[382] it's something we choose to do because we feel like it, not because we have to.

---

[381] Webster (2005).
[382] *Through the Looking-Glass* (1872).

Meat provides highly bioavailable iron, calcium, vitamin $B_{12}$ and some other nutrients. This means that those nutrients become readily available for absorption from the gut into the bloodstream, and therefore can be used in metabolic processes. Something which is not bioavailable can be present, but in a form which prevents the nutrient from being used. In practical terms, this means that vegetarians and vegans must be careful to ensure that they have adequate sources of these nutrients which are bioavailable. For example, milk and milk products contain significant amounts of bioavailable calcium and milk substitutes such as soy milk often contain added calcium salts to make sure that those who do not consume dairy products have an adequate source of calcium. A study of post-menopausal women found that absorption of calcium from soy milk fortified with calcium phosphate was similar to that from cows' milk.[383] However, there is a study of healthy men showing that calcium phosphate-fortified soy milk results in about 25% less calcium absorption than from cows' milk;[384] similar results have been obtained in young women.[385] This is an average result, and inspection of the data shows that there were quite significant differences in the level of absorption between individuals. Furthermore, the actual levels of calcium likely to be consumed and made available if soy milk is substituted for cows' milk will make up for any reduced bioavailability of calcium phosphate. There is also work showing that, despite a reduced calcium intake on a vegan diet, calcium balance and bone turnover was no different from those on a lactovegetarian diet. Thus, it seems a carefully-selected vegan diet can maintain calcium status.[386]

---

[383] Tang et al. (2010); A popular Australian soy milk, Sanitarium's *So Good*, is fortified with calcium phosphate: Sanitarium, personal communication, 20 April 2017.

[384] Heaney et al. (2000).

[385] Zhao et al. (2005). Calcium as calcium carbonate had bioavailability comparable to cows' milk.

[386] Kohlenberg-Mueller and Raschka (2003).

**Other factors influencing the choice to eat meat**

John Webster (1994) was absolutely right when he said 'we must acknowledge that we don't really consume meat, milk and cheese in order to live, but because they are among the great luxuries that determine the quality of our own lives'. Moreover, what is very important to realise is that food choices, including the choice to eat meat, are *learned*. The idea that humans eat meat because it is natural, or something our ancestors did, has no basis in fact. The foods we are exposed to as children set the scene for what we eat as adults. Seventh Day Adventists and most Buddhists are vegetarian. Jews and Muslims do not eat pig meat. Sikhs and Hindus do not eat beef. These are cultural choices. In any given social and cultural setting there are norms which will also exert pressure on food choices. Many Australians would regard a choice to not eat meat or consume dairy products as odd. Indeed such choices would in some environments be the object of ridicule. Thus, in a survey of Scottish and English vegans, Twine (2017) found that a significant majority (83%) of participants reported negative reactions from friends and family to a decision to adhere to a vegan diet.

There is a further illustration of the choice element in meat eating. If we eat meat because it provides protein and other useful nutrients, then on the face of it, there is no reason why one should not eat dogs, cats or any other animal which can provide protein for the diet. In the West, this does not happen. There is a very different perception of dogs and cows, for example. This is a consequence of the psychological framework shared by people in the West, the 'schema'; by definition this is a completely artificial construct,[387] as is the choice to eat meat *per se*.

In the main, people do not want to associate the item of food they are eating with the animal it came from. No doubt this in part accounts for the rise in popularity of the fast food burgers, rolls and so on, which bear no resemblance to the source animal. As Joy says, it is rare these

---

[387] Joy (2016).

days to be served the whole head of an animal for that reason.[388] The meat producing industry is very aware of this, and has gone to a huge amount of trouble and expense to dissociate the identity of the animal from the food on the plate.[389]

Why then do most humans like to eat meat? The short answer is because that is what they are brought up to do and what society expects them to do. Peter Singer, in *Animal Liberation*, gave a one word answer to the question: 'habit'. Thus the influence of parents on the development of childrens' meat eating habits is substantial.[390] Surveys have indicated that many people who eat meat do so because they think meat has a 'good taste'.[391] Eating meat is an acquired taste and coping with the emotional stress involved in knowing you are eating a bit of an animal which has been killed so you can eat it comes about by the process of 'psychic numbing', which itself is acquired, not innate.[392] Bastian et al. (2012) identified another way of coping with this paradox. They found that people regarded animals they ate as having lower mental capacities than those they didn't eat. But this attitude is compounded by the fact that Australians in general have little understanding of the production processes involved in generating their animal-based food (Chen, 2016).

Of course the corollary to all of this is that going back as far as 2,500 years ago, people (even then) were choosing not to eat meat on ethical grounds.[393] That said, one of the arguments often mounted in favour of eating meat is that it is 'natural' and humans have been doing it for millenia. This is intellectually feeble, as the ancestors of the human race did all sorts of things which they would have thought as 'natural', including infanticide, murder, rape and cannibalism, to name but a few.

---

388 Joy (2016).
389 see Plous (2003).
390 Chen (2016).
391 eg Mullee et al.(2017).
392 Joy (2016).
393 Joy (2016).

Nobody in their right mind would justify those activities on the grounds that 'we've always done it'.[394]

It is very interesting that, while there is a very long way to go, many commercial ventures have entered the area of non-meat 'meat alternatives'. Many of the technologies employed use plant material, but there are also significant efforts to produce meat-like foods from meat cells grown in culture.[395]

## Why not eat meat?

'Vegetarianism is harmless enough, though it is apt to fill a man with wind and self-righteousness', said Robert Hutchison to the British Medical Association in 1930.[396] The implication is that not eating meat is of no benefit. Today, it is fair to say there are many reasons to seriously question the wisdom of eating meat (leaving aside the huge negative impact of meat-eating on animal welfare). Growing animals to kill them to eat contributes substantially to the level of atmospheric greenhouse gases. Reduction in meat consumption is predicted to ease pressure on land use and will greatly reduce diet-related mortality, particularly if there is a corresponding increase in fruit and vegetable intake.[397]

## Over-eating

In the developed world many people eat too much. One of the reasons for this is that the relative cost of food which is energy-dense has decreased. There is also a greater reliance on highly-processed and palatable 'convenience foods'. The most obvious result of this over-consumption is obesity. In 2014-15, 63% of Australians were overweight or obese.[398] The obesity rate in children is approaching 30%. These are huge increases which have occurred in recent years. Obesity has serious

---

[394] Joy (2016), 106
[395] see Goodfellow (2015).
[396] see Gale et al. (2006).
[397] Springmann et al.(2016).
[398] ABS (2015).

consequences, such as greatly increasing the likelihood of Type 2 (insulin-independent) diabetes.[399] In 2014-15, one million Australians had Type 2 diabetes.[400] The upshot is that it is probable that today's generation of children will be the first to have a life expectancy lower than their parents.[401]

The 2016 survey of food group consumption from the Australian Bureau of Statistics (which uses data collected in 2011-12)[402] indicates that over-consumption of food generally is not associated with over-consumption of meat. Only 14% of those surveyed had meat intakes equaling or exceeding the current dietary recommendations.[403] This was highly age-dependent: older people (51-70) were far likelier to meet recommended intakes (about 30%) while only 18% of males and 5% of females in the 19-50 age group met or exceeded the recommendations. Red meat and poultry together made up 68% of consumption, while all red meat (which included pork) contributed 38%. The dietary guidelines say in effect that, because of this seemingly low intake, compared to the recommendations, people should eat more meat.

---

[399] Insulin is a hormone secreted by the pancreas. Insulin levels go up as blood glucose levels rise, and the effect of the insulin is to allow cells to absorb glucose. In Type 2 diabetes, cells become resistant to insulin, so glucose is poorly absorbed into the cells, so that blood glucose rises. The maintained increase in blood glucose is what causes the damaging consequences of diabetes: increased risk of stroke and blindness, as well as cardiovascular disease. Other consequences of obesity include increased risk of cardiovascular disease, hypertension, some cancers, reproductive disorders as well as mental disease such as depression: NHMRC (2013).

[400] ABS (2015),

[401] NHMRC (2013).

[402] The data come from the National Nutrition and Physical Activity Survey, published by the Australian Bureau of Statistics (cat no 4364.0.55.007).

[403] The recommendations vary somewhat depending on age, but for adults, the recommended intake is roughly 3 serves per day; a serve of lean red meat is 65g, while a serve of poultry is 80g.

I do not believe these survey figures; they may be a considerable under-estimation of meat intake. The ABARES 2016 report on Australian Commodities shows *apparent* consumption per person for 2015 as 76g/day for beef and veal,[404] 76g/day for pork[405] and 124g/day for chicken.[406] These figures are calculated on the basis of how much of these meats are produced, minus exports, plus imports, although they do not consider wastage. I have calculated daily intake by reference to the Australian population at the end of 2015, which was 23,871,000.[407] This indicates strongly that the consumption of meat is much greater than indicated by the dietary survey and is very much in excess of the recommended intake – particularly as the calculation I have made makes no allowance for age; that population number represents the entire population, of all ages. Note, however, that this calculation makes no allowance for food which is bought and then thrown away, which may be a considerable amount. Given that the dietary guidelines recommend lower meat consumption for children, the apparent consumption figures from the ABARES report point to a serious under-estimate of consumption in the nutrition survey. The important message here is that any call for increased meat consumption based on the 2016 survey is in all likelihood based on wrong data. The dietary guidelines make such a recommendation.

I note in passing that the dietary guidelines call for a 40% increase in fish consumption. This is likely to be unsustainable without an increase in the amount of imported fish. But this recommendation may again be based on faulty data. It says that the survey shows that weekly consumption of fish is 168g/week for men, and 119g/week for women. But a recent IBIS survey indicates that seafood consumption is 19kg per

---

[404] 661kt per annum.

[405] 27.9kg per person per annum.

[406] 1,084kt per annum.

[407] Australian Bureau of Statistics *Australian Demographic Statistics* (cat no 3101.0).

person per year.[408] This corresponds to 365g/person per week, which is more than double the consumption indicated by the survey.

There is an urban myth (which is more prevalent in rural parts, in my view) that a vegetarian or vegan diet is inadequate. For example, it is often said that animal protein must be consumed for normal brain function. This is not true. The Australian Dietary Guidelines say:

> *'Appropriately planned vegetarian diets, including total vegetarian or vegan diets, are healthy and nutritionally adequate...those following a vegan diet should choose foods to ensure adequate intake of iron and zinc and to optimise the absorption and bioavailability of iron, zinc and calcium. Supplementation of vitamin $B_{12}$ may be required for people with strict vegan dietary patterns.'[409]*

### The positive effects of eating vegetables and fruit

Not only is a vegetarian or vegan diet adequate, but there is convincing evidence, cited in the national dietary guidelines, that eating 'plenty of vegetables' has positive health benefits, such as protecting against cardiovascular disease. The guidelines say there is 'strengthened evidence' of the beneficial effects of intake of various non-starchy vegetables in reducing risk of some cancers.[410] Furthermore, there is recent evidence that consuming vegetables is associated with a reduced

---

[408] IBISWorld (15 December 2015) *Soaring seafood consumption fails to deliver significant growth for Australia's fishing and aquaculture industries.* www.ibisworld.com.au/media/2015/12/14/soaring-seafood-consumption-fails-to-deliver-significant-growth-for-australias-fishing-and-aquaculture-industries/.

[409] NHMRC (2013).

[410] NHMRC (2013); there is suggestive evidence that consuming vegetables reduces the risk of oral and nasopharyngeal cancers; there is some evidence of reduced risk of other alimentary cancers, such as oesophageal cancer; there is some evidence that consumption of tomatoes (which contain lycopenes) reduces the risk of prostate cancer; there is tenuous evidence regarding colorectal cancer and intake of non-starchy vegetables; even lung cancer risk may be reduced by consumption of vegetables containing carotenoids.

risk of weight gain. The same can be said of fruit consumption. The most recent dietary guidelines say that the evidence of health advantages of fruit consumption has 'strengthened considerably recently'.[411] There is a probability that eating fruit reduces the risk of coronary heart disease. Regarding cancers, there is emerging evidence for positive effects of fruit consumption on the risk of alimentary tract cancer. What is also clear is that eating fruit and vegetables in reasonable quantities does not *increase* the risk of cancers.

What is particularly fascinating about the most recent scientific data regarding vegetable and fruit intake is that there is growing evidence that various components of these foods may have positive effects. For example, anti-oxidants such as vitamins C and E, and other phytochemicals, may have the effect of ultimately reducing the deposition of plaques in blood vessels. This will have the effect of preventing many serious cardiovascular conditions, such as stroke and blockage of coronary arteries.

Given all this, the current Australian dietary guidelines recommend consuming at least 375g of vegetables and 300g of fruit per day. The guidelines point out that the significant nutrient profile of legumes could benefit all Australians – that is, not just vegetarians and vegans.

The other vegetable-based food with positive health benefits is the grain (ie mostly wholegrain) and high cereal fibre food group. Consumption of these foods is associated with reduced risk of cardiovascular disease, type 2 diabetes and excess weight gain.[412] There is also some recent evidence supporting the idea that the risk of colorectal cancer is reduced by eating high fibre cereals.

Surveys of consumption show that less than 4% of Australians meet the vegetable consumption guidelines; for children, it is less than 1%.[413]

---

[411] NHMRC (2013).
[412] NHMRC (2013).
[413] ABS (2016).

## The negative effects of eating meat

Springmann and colleagues have said decreasing consumption of red meat and increasing consumption of fruits and vegetables, coupled with reductions in total energy intake, could result in reductions in premature mortality of 6-10%.[414] Processed and cured meats are a particular problem. They can be high in added salt and saturated fat, both of which are bad for one's health.[415] One particular risk with processed and cured meats is they contain chemicals which may generate cancer-causing molecules, such as N-nitroso compounds. These have been suggested as a possible link between red meat consumption and colorectal cancer.[416]

Replacing saturated fat with monounsaturated and polyunsaturated fats is associated with improved blood lipid profiles and reduced risk of cardiovascular disease. The current dietary guidelines make reference to the possibility that saturated fats in meat may be a risk factor for cardiovascular disease. However, they note that this risk may not be present when lean meat is consumed.

The Australian dietary guidelines published in 2013 say: 'since the 2003 edition of the dietary guidelines, the evidence linking meat consumption and increased risk of disease has strengthened in some areas and remain unclear in others'.[417] For example, the guidelines say there have not been sufficient studies investigating the relationships between consumption of meat, type 2 diabetes and excess weight to draw any conclusions. However, there is evidence of a probable association between consumption of red meat and increased risk of colorectal cancer. There is suggestive evidence regarding increased risk of renal cancer, and suggestive evidence of no association between

---

[414] Springmann et al.(2016).
[415] NHMRC (2013).
[416] NHMRC (2013); Bouvard et al.(2015).
[417] NHMRC (2013). It appears the problem arises because of varying definitions of what is 'meat' in the studies. Thus, some studies include processed meats, or define 'red meat' differently.

meat consumption and increased risk of bladder, prostate and pancreatic cancer.

Even though more and more national nutritional guidelines include warnings about the health consequences of (over-) eating meat, it is quite likely that many people who do eat meat do not think there are any risks involved.[418] This represents a failure of governments to properly educate people – probably motivated by a wish not to upset farmers.

## Alternatives to meat

The proportion of vegetarians in Australia has risen in recent years, to 1.7 million (or nearly 10% of the population) in 2016. In New South Wales there has been a 30% increase in the number of people saying they are vegetarian.[419] It seems that concern for health and wellbeing (as well as ethical concerns about animals) is a major driver of the choice.[420] The counter to that is being vegan or vegetarian is probably still regarded by many in the community an unusual choice, with all the associated social stigma.[421] Having said that, there is a strong bias towards females being vegetarians; there is also evidence that females who eat meat are more apologetic about it, and use indirect strategies, such as mentally dissociating animals from food.[422]

The Australian dietary guidelines say firmly that non-meat foods can be an adequate source of all the nutrients which are also provided by meat. So, nuts and seeds are energy-rich, contain protein and dietary fibre, and significant levels of unsaturated fatty acids and micronutrients such as folate, vitamin E, selenium, magnesium and other minerals. Likewise,

---

[418] Mullee et al.(2017).

[419] Roy Morgan Research (2016) *The slow but steady rise of vegetarianism in Australia.*

[420] Roy Morgan Research (2013) *Meat-free, health conscious and a little bit anxious: Australia's vegetarians.*

[421] Chen (2012). Mullee et al.(2016) report that 25% of respondents in a Belgian survey believed that eating vegetarian food is unhealthy.

[422] Cornish et al. (2016).

the guidelines are clear that lentils, tofu and other foods based on beans or legumes are 'a valuable and cost-efficient source of protein, iron, some essential fatty acids, soluble and insoluble dietary fibre and micronutrients'.[423]

Even the meat industry is monitoring trends regarding meat eating closely.[424] It appears that recent research indicates that 28% of Australian meat eaters may be intending to reduce the amount of meat they consume. Concerns about animal welfare are a major driver of this seeming change.

There is increasing availablity of remarkably palatable plant-sourced meat alternatives. Indeed, the Chief Executive Officer of Tyson Foods, one of the biggest meat producers in the USA, recently alluded to a meatless food future. Apparently Tyson Foods has bought a small stake in an enterprise called Beyond Meat, which produces meat substitutes based on plant material.[425] Impossible Foods in the US has raised over $180 million from well known investors, including Google and Bill Gates. Commentators have expressed the view that burgers made using novel technology will within a few years have captured a significant part of the market.[426]

Technology enabling the production of large numbers of cells from 'immortalised' cell lines has been available for many decades now. Most recently, this has enabled the development of cultured meat, which exploits the proliferative properties of embryonic muscle cells. Although this is some way from making a real commercial impact, and is still reliant on the use of foetal calf serum as a growth medium,[427] it is nevertheless coming close to reality. A Committee of the US National

[423] NHMRC (2013).
[424] Goodwin (2016) Red meat processors look closely at changing consumer patterns. *Farm Online*
[425] Fox Business, 7 March 2017; see www.beyondmeat.com.
[426] James Nason *Plant-based burgers could take a big bite from beef, expert warns*. Beef Central 19 May 2017
[427] Dilworth and McGregor (2015).

Academies of Sciences, Engineering and Medicine has said it 'expects to see growth in the number and market acceptance of such food products as they are being marketed as more sustainable and cruelty-free'.[428] Analyses have shown that, compared to normal meat production, this technology will involve less energy use (except when compared to chicken meat), lower greenhouse gas production, less water use and almost no land use.[429]

**Not eating meat: overview**

The final statement should go to the US Academy of Nutrition and Dietetics:

> *'It is the position of the Academy of Nutrition and Dietetics that appropriately planned vegetarian, including vegan, diets are healthful, nutritionally adequate, and may provide health benefits for the prevention and treatment of certain diseases. These diets are appropriate for all stages of the life cycle, including pregnancy, lactation, infancy, childhood, adolescence, older adulthood and for athletes... Vegetarians and vegans are at reduced risk of certain health conditions, including ischemic heart disease, type 2 diabetes, hypertension, certain types of cancer and obesity. Low intake of saturated fat and high intakes of vegetables, fruits, whole grains, legumes, soy products, nuts and seeds (all rich in fiber and phytochemicals) are characteristics of vegetarian and vegan diets that produce lower total and low-density lipoprotein cholesterol levels and better serum glucose control. These factors contribute to reduction of chronic disease'.[430]*

One of the key phrases in this statement is 'appropriately planned'. Because meat contains several essential nutrients which are not found

---

[428] Committee on future biotechnology products and opportunities to enhance capabilities of the biotechnology regulatory system (2017) *Preparing for future products of biotechnology.*
[429] Tuomisto and Joost Teixeira de Mattos (2011).
[430] Melina et al. (2016).

in many vegetables, it is important to make sure that a vegetarian or vegan diet contains sources of those nutrients. As I have already mentioned, there must be an adequate source of calcium, which could be a fortified non-dairy milk. Vitamin $B_{12}$ can be sourced in various fortified foods, such as breakfast cereals and soy milks. Iron and zinc are found in good quantities in legumes, tofu and whole grains. Omega-3 fatty acids are present in canola oil and walnuts, amongst other sources.

## Marketing meat

One must never forget that those who profit from growing and killing animals for food are the 'biggest economic beneficiaries from the marginalisation of voices promoting animal rights.'[431] I believe, however, that the animal use industry portrayal of those concerned with animal welfare as an unhinged minority has had its day. Those concerned with animal welfare are now a very substantial proportion of their customers. This means of course that the meat marketers have to adopt more subtle approaches to persuading people to keep consuming their product.

The meat industry in Australia has been very clever in the marketing of its product. For example it has portrayed meat as being something associated with masculinity[432] and in a most effective (but demonstrably dishonest) advertising campaign, featuring well-known actor Sam Neill, something that is responsible for the evolution of human intellectual ability. Leading social scientists have for years pointed to the obvious purported connection between perceived virility and meat-eating.[433] The association with masculinity is probably quite real – Norwegian soldiers encouraged to reduce meat consumption were reluctant to do so because of meat's perceived association with masculinity.[434]

---

[431] Pendergrast (2015).
[432] Chen (2012).
[433] see Lund et al. (2016).
[434] Kildal and Syse (2017).

Even today there are those who maintain that human ancestors ate meat, therefore it makes sense for modern humans to eat meat. Pete Evans and his paleo diet is one example. There is no evidence to support this. As Plous (2002) has said, 'the anthropological and historical record suggests that the earlier hominids were not prodigious hunters, but rather were limited to opportunistic scavenging of carcass remnants abandoned by carnivores'. In any case, what the ancestors of humanity did is beside the point. The question is what should we eat now.

Aesthetic objections to the awful processes involved in production of meat from animals have been around for some time. Henry Salt was one such early advocate of vegetarianism, relying on aesthetic arguments.[435] As one would expect given the strong tendency of people to dissociate the idea of an actual animal from the meat they eat, images of animals on meat packages in supermarkets are either absent or stylized.[436] The place where animals are kept – the farm – is likewise presented in heavily censored imagery; 'in the symbolic language of the Australian supermarket, farmers and farms are depicted as clean, largely free of animals, and somewhat quaint.'[437] The art of preparation of many meat dishes has emphasised changing the form of the ingredients so as not to be recognisably from an animal. The killing of animals is never mentioned.[438] Consistent with this, Anderson and Barrett (2016) found that pairing meat samples to be eaten with descriptions of animals raised on factory farms (compared to extensive farms) resulted in a different eating experience for survey participants. Factory farmed meat samples were said to taste more salty and greasy, and participants consumed less of it.

Meat and Livestock Australia's Global Tracker study has shown that in 2016, 24% of Australian males who prepare meals (and are over the age of 18 years) believe that beef or lamb consumption should be limited to

---

[435] see Holdier (2016).
[436] Webster (1994); Chen (2012).
[437] Chen (2012).
[438] Hoogland et al. (2005).

avoid possible health problems. This has led to an advertising campaign ('the Trinity Experiment') designed to 'highlight that a healthy balanced diet featuring beef and lamb helps humankind be the best it can be'.[439]

The emphasis on health is clearly something the industry thinks is working for them, with the latest beef campaign from Meat and Livestock Australia underscoring the utility of beef as a source of iron for women.[440]

In my view, it is of concern that influential and popular cooking programmes such as *My Kitchen Rules* and *Masterchef* very rarely feature vegetarian meals.

## Meat eating and the environment, and other risks
*'Buy land, they're not making it anymore'*.[441]

Raising animals involves the devouring and ruination of land. Eventually, growing animals on land to supply food will simply stop working. There won't be enough land, or what's left will be polluted and unusable, or both.

So, although this is ostensibly nothing to do with the welfare of farmed animals,[442] there is no doubt that there are huge environmental costs of eating. Meat production is one of the major contributors to global environmental degradation. Livestock raised for meat use 30% of the world's land and 8% of its fresh water. Livestock production is responsible for much deforestation and removal of wildlife habitats.

Ruminant livestock, such as cattle and sheep, produce significant amounts of the greenhouse gases responsible for global warming.

---

[439] MLA nutrition campaigns: www.mla.com.au/marketing-beef-and-lamb/domestic-marketing/nutrition-campaigns/
[440] www.mla.com.au/marketing-beef-and-lamb/domestic-marketing/beef-campaigns
[441] Mark Twain, as quoted by Raworth (2017).
[442] Obviously wild animals suffer considerably as a result of land clearing for agricultural use.

Livestock production is responsible for 18% of greenhouse gases.[443] The main gas produced is methane, which is said to be 25 times 'worse' than carbon dioxide as a greenhouse gas. The production of livestock is also environmentally costly in terms of water, land and fertiliser use. It is notable, however, that production of dairy products, poultry, pork and eggs is significantly less costly in terms of these factors than beef production.[444]

Consumption of chicken meat is increasing rapidly. Apart from the obvious animal welfare issues, there are other, perhaps not so obvious problems associated with increased reliance on chicken meat. For example, there has recently been an outbreak of 'bird flu' (avian influenza) strain H5N8 in the UK, which resulted in mandatory indoor housing for all poultry (to minimise contact with wild birds carrying the virus). While this particular strain of 'bird flu' is considered a low risk for humans, it is just a matter of time before strains evolve which are problematic for human health. The risks of having huge numbers of poultry which can become infected are obvious. Intensive poultry farms are nothing more or less than enormous incubators for any bird virus that happens to get in.

Resistance to antibiotics is a major threat to the effective treatment of bacterial infections;[445] the threat is growing.[446] Direct use of antibiotics in people is a major contributor to this problem, but use of antibiotics in food animals is also thought to play an important part. The issue relates not only to human health, but also to animal health and the productivity of the animal food industry.

The World Health Organisation has recently stated that antibiotics are used in greater quantities in healthy food-producing animals than in the

---

[443] FAO (2006).
[444] Tuomisto and Mattos (2011); Eshel et al. (2014).
[445] Barton (2000).
[446] Collignon (2015).

treatment of disease in human patients.[447] Professor Peter Collignon of the Australian National University believes that 80% or more of the world usage of antibiotics is for use in food animals, although he points out that proper usage data is lacking.[448] Antibiotics are often used in these animals as growth promoters, whereby they are given to ostensibly healthy animals, usually in their food or water. The food animal industry has always maintained that antibiotic use is associated with improved growth rate and feed conversion efficiency.[449] Professor Collignon argues that the claimed growth promotion and prophylaxis effects are 'marginal', and there have not been well controlled studies to back the belief that antibiotics produce these effects.[450]

The antibiotics used in food animals can be the same as those used in human medicine, and this widespread use of large quantities of antibiotics, whether it be in humans or animals, carries with it the risk of emergence of strains of antibiotic-resistant bacteria. These drug-resistant bacteria present an obvious threat to human health, as people infected with such strains may not respond to treatment with antibiotics, with potentially lethal consequences.[451] This is not relevant only to bacteria which infect both animals and people, as animal-specific bacteria which become drug-resistant have the potential to spread genes for drug resistance (as 'plasmids', or little mobile DNA sequences) to human bacteria.[452] The problem of antibiotic resistance

---

[447] World Health Organization (2012) *The evolving threat of antimicrobial resistance – options for action*.

[448] Collignon (2015).

[449] Joint Export Advisory Committee on Antibiotic Resistance (1999) *The use of antibiotics in food-producing animals: antibiotic-resistant bacteria in animals and humans*.

[450] Collignon (2012); (2004).

[451] Drug resistance may lead to increased frequency of treatment failure, increased severity of infection, prolonged duration of illness, increased frequency of bloodstream infection, increased hospitalization or increased mortality: Heuer et al. (2009).

[452] Note that drug-resistance genes are often complex and have probably been in the environment for many years (possibly billions), albeit at low levels.

is exacerbated by a dramatic decrease in pharmaceutical industry research directed towards production of new antibiotics resulting in a dramatic reduction in registration of new antibiotics.[453] This has happened simply because it is no longer very profitable to develop antibiotics.

It is not only the use of antibacterials in farm animals which may be contributing to the problem of drug resistance. Use of antimicrobial agents in farmed fish has resulted in the emergence of antimicrobial-resistant bacteria in fish and other aquatic animals. These drug resistant bacteria are also present in the aquatic environment.[454] Arguably, the use of these drugs in fish is associated with the risks involved with use of antibiotics in farm animals.

Another possible source of risk is that of accumulation of antibiotics in the environment, including soil, for example where manure from animals treated with antibiotics is applied as fertilizer.[455]

The WHO has concluded *"it is clear that action is needed to reduce the use of antibiotics in food animals."*[456]

Data for antimicrobial use in Australian animals up to 2010 shows that in a five-year period, 587 tonnes were used. Ninety-eight per cent of these drugs were used in farm animals. Four percent of this usage was said to be for growth promotion. Fifty percent or so of the drug use was related to the control of coccidiosis in chickens – coccidiostats are not 'antibiotics' in the strict sense, so this use can be discounted.[457] In Australia, until now there has been a lack of clarity about how often

---

[453] Department of Health / Department of Agriculture (2015) *Responding to the threat of antimicrobial resistance*. See also Shaban et al. (2014).

[454] Shaban et al. (2014).

[455] Jechalke et al. (2014).

[456] World Health Organization (2012) *The evolving threat of antimicrobial resistance – options for action*.

[457] Department of Health (2015) *Responding to the threat of antimicrobial resistance*.

antibiotics are given to farm animals. That may be about to change, with the release in November 2016 of a National Antimicrobial Resistance Strategy, which will (amongst other things) involve a new surveillance system designed to monitor antibiotic use in the agriculture sector.[458] This will include programmes to determine the prevalence of antimicrobial resistance in food animals and in animal-derived food. The strategy refers to the 'One Health' concept, which recognises that human, animal and ecosystem health are closely linked. It also acknowledges there is increasing evidence pointing to antibiotic use in agriculture as contributing to the emergence, persistence and spread of resistant bacteria. However, it notes that 'the impact of antimicrobial usage in agriculture in Australia is not well understood'. The increasing importance of this issue can be seen by the fact that it is being cited and analysed by those responsible for assessing risks to investors. The view is that the agriculture industry will have to lift its game on matters of this sort if investors are to continue risking their money in the animal farming business.[459]

In 2006 the Expert Advisory Group on Antimicrobial Resistance updated its report rating the importance of antimicrobials for human use.[460] This provides a useful indicator of the antimicrobials whose use in animals ought to be restricted. The Australian Pesticides and Veterinary Medicines Authority (APVMA) is responsible for the authorisation of use of antibiotics in food animals. The drugs are used essentially in three ways: (1) antimicrobial use for treatment of disease, or (2) for prophylactic use to prevent the development of disease, which is

---

[458] see www.health.gov.au/internet/main/publishing.nsf/Content/ohp-amr.htm. I am grateful to Associate Professor Thomas Gottlieb of Sydney University for bringing this to my attention.
[459] AMP Capital (April 2017) *Is factory farming making us sick? Human resistance to antibiotics: an earnings risk for the global food and beverage sector.*
[460] see appendix reproducing the EAGAR importance ratings: Australian Pesticides and Veterinary Medicines Authority (2014) *Quantity of antimicrobial products sold for veterinary use in Australia.*

restricted to use 'under the direction of a veterinarian' and use for growth promotion (3), which is in essence unrestricted. The potential for antimicrobial resistance is a criterion for registration by APVMA of a product for use in food animals.[461] However, as of April 2017, there is no requirement for postmarketing surveillance of resistance for newly-registered antibiotics in humans or animals. This is despite the fact that, since 2004, other valuable classes of antibiotics which are used in humans have also been approved for animal use. However, only one third generation cephalosporin has been approved for use in animals, and it seems its actual use is quite small.

A 2006 survey found antibiotics rated as 'high importance' were not widely used in the Australian pig industry and that many of the antibiotics which were used were rated as being of 'low importance' for human health.[462] Even so, it is of concern that this survey found that the important third generation cephalosporin ceftiofur was used in about 25% of herds sampled. Current data is urgently needed.

General observations of antibiotic use in cattle in countries where there is a high level of intensive confinement cannot be applied uncritically to the Australian position. The majority of cattle in this country are not kept in intensive facilities. Furthermore, it may be that effective quarantine measures have so far prevented the entry into Australia of some antimicrobial-resistant bacteria (eg some multi-drug resistant non-typhoidal *Salmonella*).[463] Another important consideration is that many antibiotics used in animals have no direct equivalent in human medicine.[464]

However, there are indications that the problem of antibiotic resistance is increasing in Australia. Thus, the Australian Antibiotic Resistance Group has reported that resistance to methicillin in *Staphylococcus*

---

[461] see http://www.apvma.gov.au/node/1013.
[462] Jordan et al. (2009).
[463] Shaban et al. (2014).
[464] Shaban et al. (2014).

*aureus* bacteraemia isolates was about 19% in 2013, significantly higher than the level reported in most European countries.[465]

## Handling, transport and control of animals

Transportation of animals from the location where they have been kept to a slaughterhouse can be associated with poor welfare due to stress, starvation, trauma and extremes of heat and cold. It seems that the welfare problems associated with animal transport have increased because of a reduction in the number of slaughter facilities through industry consolidation. This is especially true in remote areas of northern Australia,[466] a situation made worse by the effect of live export in making local processing less economically viable. Jed Goodfellow (2015) notes that in 2010, nearly 750,000 sheep and 80,000 cattle were transported the large distance from Western Australia to abattoirs in eastern Australia.

Handling, loading and transport are especially stressful times for animals, just because of the disruption of their normal routines and the shock of the new. Clearly, handling animals requires skill and knowledge; an experienced and sympathetic stockperson can mean the difference between good welfare and bad welfare. Also, it is not just welfare which is an issue, as highly stressed animals which need to be transported significant distances will end up producing meat of lower quality. Transport of pigs and poultry can be associated with serious temperature control issues, as these animals cannot regulate heat loss by sweating.[467]

The journey to the slaughterhouse may be interrupted by the animal passing through a market or saleyard. In Australia, transport is usually by land, although there are some sea journeys (for example from Tasmania). For shorter journeys, it may be necessary to withhold feed and water so that the animals do not produce significant quantities of

---

[465] see http://www.agargroup.org.
[466] Goodfellow (2015).
[467] Webster (2005).

urine and faeces while on the transport vehicle. Loading and unloading represent stages in the process where there are clear risks of injury.[468]

The transport of chickens for slaughter is likely to be particularly traumatic. For caged chickens, a number of birds are grabbed and pulled out of the cage, then passed to another person who may carry two to five birds held by a leg, upside down, to a crate for transport. This will in all likelihood result in broken bones. Broom and Fraser (2007) refer to one study which found 24% of hens had broken bones after handling.

Animals being driven on a vehicle brace themselves to avoid being thrown around, and do not brace themselves against other animals. They are disturbed by too much movement or too high a stocking density.[469] Reducing the height of decks on transport vehicles may also reduce the efficiency of ventilation.

There have been some improvements in the design of races and laneways for moving animals to and from transport vehicles. Broom and Fraser (2007) describe the work of Grandin, who has identified particular problems associated with badly designed races. Thus, cattle will baulk at dark areas or areas of sharp lighting contrast. Angular turns can also be problematical.[470]

## Killing animals to eat – slaughter

The modern western slaughterhouse is an exercise in denial of reality. As with other aspects of raising and killing animals for food, euphemisms abound. The slaughterhouse or abattoir is now the 'processing plant'. The operators of the plants do not want people to see what goes on there, and probably the consumers of the product in plastic packs at the supermarket don't really want to know. No matter what farmers and animal users might say about people needing to know where their food comes from, I see no future in tourist trips around

---

[468] Broom and Fraser (2007).
[469] Broom and Fraser (2007).
[470] Grandin (2013).

abattoirs. Slaughterhouses are designed to keep the nastiness away from public view, and no sane person would pretend that slaughterhouses are pleasant places. Furthermore, there is plenty of evidence to suggest that in many cases slaughter of animals is carried out in a callous and vicious manner.[471] There is little doubt that in the real world of the slaughterhouse, people involved in handling and killing animals are quite likely to become brutal.[472] Recent footage obtained from two Tasmanian abattoirs show very young calves (bobby calves) being abused and thrown into a restrainer, and in another establishment, pigs which had been inadequately stunned (so were conscious when they had their throats slit). There are plenty of other examples. It does seem to me that much of what is said about the need for humane practices in slaughterhouses is looking for the impossible. The reality is appalling and the unfortunate people who have to work there must suffer a serious psychological impact from doing what they do. It is hardly surprising that there is so much evidence of cruelty.

Professor John Webster is of the view that, while humans are a 'sufficiently sentient species to be aware of and so fear death', this may not necessarily be the same for other animal species. He believes that possibly primates and elephants may experience the concept of death in ways similar to humans, but other species (eg sheep, cattle) are 'unconcerned' when a member of their species is killed in front of them. He therefore concludes that the concept of death is not a welfare problem, and it follows that it is not cruel to kill an animal if it can be done without causing pain, fear or any other form of distress.

There are two main ways in which growing animals for slaughter are regarded. Animal welfare organisations, such as the various RPSCAs, regard 'humane' slaughter of animals as acceptable. This is very much the view of the average member of the public. The alternative view is that killing animals to eat them (or in any other way exploit them) is

---

[471] Dalziell and Wadiwei (2017).
[472] see Fitzgerald et al.(2009).

wrong.[473] However, it is blindingly obvious that if reports of cruelty in slaughterhouses are framed according to the second view, they will not get media coverage.[474]

The core concept in slaughter is that it should be 'humane'.[475] This widely-used word is not formally defined, but is usually taken to be associated with all the usual comforting words about how animals should be treated. Legislation governing the licensing of abattoirs incorporates compliance with one or other slaughter code as a condition of the licence. The code most usually referenced is the Australian Standard for the Hygienic Production and Transportation of Meat and Meat Products for Human Consumption (AS4696:2007). This code requires that animals must be slaughtered in a way that prevents unnecessary injury, pain and suffering and causes them 'the least practicable disturbance'. It is generally thought that the key to 'humane' slaughter is that animals should be stunned before they are killed.[476] The killing involves cutting major blood vessels, usually those in the neck, after which the dying animal is hoisted up to allow blood to drain out. Stunning can use various techniques, the two major ones being percussive stunning and electrical stunning.[477] Percussive stunning involves a gun which shoots a tethered projectile (a 'captive bolt') to either penetrate the skull, or (using a mushroom shaped bolt) to deliver a huge blow to the skull, and thereby cause a massive shock to the brain

---

[473] Pendergrast (2015), 101.

[474] Pendergrast (2015), 116.

[475] See Grandin (2013). The law in Australia governing slaughter mirrors other law relating to animal welfare. It is inconsistent and in the main inadequate. Slaughter of animals for meat for export is governed by the *Export Control Act 1982* and relevant subsidiary legislation. States and Territories law includes the *Food Regulation 2015* (NSW), *Food Production (Safety) Regulation 2014* (Qld), *Primary Produce (Food Safety Schemes) (Meat Industry) Regulations 2006* (SA), *Meat Industry Act 1993* (Vic) and *Western Australian Meat Industry Authority Act 1976* (WA). All of these require abattoirs to be licensed.

[476] This principle is abandoned when the animal is slaughtered according to religious principles that demand the animal be conscious when it is killed.

[477] see Terlouw et al.(2016) for a detailed review.

of the animal. This causes loss of consciousness, primarily because of brain damage caused by the shock wave. Poor placement of the stunning pistol may result in the animal being partially or fully conscious. Electrical stunning uses two electrodes placed either side of the brain which delivers sufficient electrical current to induce an epileptic seizure, during which the animal is entirely unconscious. In non-penetrating captive bolt stunning and electrical stunning the unconsciousness is not permanent. For example, sheep and pigs begin to regain consciousness about 40 seconds after the stun. This means that the killing (so-called 'sticking') must be complete within that time frame after the stun. This raises another question, which is the length of time it takes for an animal to die after its blood vessels have been cut. That is determined by the length of time it takes for the blood supply to the brain to cease. With sheep, severing both carotid arteries will result in death of all animals within 20 seconds. However, in cattle, the vertebral arteries, as well as the carotid arteries, carry a significant amount of blood from the heart to the brain. This means that loss of brain function after cutting both carotid arteries can take up to two minutes. WIth cattle, there can also be complications caused by resealing of artery ends after the cut. This can be minimised by appropriate positioning of the head and neck.[478]

On the ground, it is apparent that there can be significant and regular problems with stunning and sticking procedures. Atkinson et al (2013) found in a study of Swedish slaughterhouses that nearly 13% of cattle were stunned inadequately, while stun to stick times had a mean value of 105 seconds, but could be as long as 140 seconds or thereabouts.

In poultry stunning, the birds are suspended upside down from metal shackles, and then dipped in a water bath into which is passed (via an electrode) an electric charge, which then passes through the shackles into the bird, thereby stunning the brain and also stopping the heart. In larger abattoirs, pigs are often stunned by putting them in a pit which

---

[478] see Grandin (2013).

has been filled with carbon dioxide. Some have reported that pigs quietly lose consciousness, while others have said that some animals struggle violently and try to climb out of the pit. Recent work has shown that the so-called 'stress hormone', cortisol, is elevated about ten-fold in young pigs subjected to increased levels of carbon dioxide; all animals showed behaviours indicative of stress, such as escape attempts.[479] It may be that animals which do panic are those with a particular genetic predisposition.[480] Whatever the situation, stunning animals with carbon dioxide is not good enough. Better, but more expensive systems, such as those using argon, are available.

Treatment of animals in abattoirs involves a complex of systems and treatments, all of which need to be considered in the context of their effect on the animal. Proper design of walkways, chutes and ramps and restraining devices (such as conveyer belts and V-belts) can hugely decrease stress levels and difficulties associated with moving animals. Use of electric prods should be minimised. All of this has obvious benefits for the animals, but also increases the efficiency of the slaughter process, thereby benefitting the plant's operators. Whatever stunning method is used, it is critical that operators should be able to properly assess whether an animal has lost consciousness. Finally, all of this must be continually assessed and audited in a meaningful way. The work of Temple Grandin has been instrumental in improving things in US abattoirs and represents a model which should be considered and followed.[481]

Under Australian law, those slaughtering animals for consumption by people of the Jewish or Muslim faiths can do so without having to stun the animals first.[482] Arguments have often been put that this is acceptable on welfare grounds because a cut to the neck with a sharp

---

[479] Sutherland et al. (2017).

[480] Grandin (2013).

[481] see Grandin (2013).

[482] Note that some interpreters of Islamic law accept non-penetrating stunning, while others don't: see Fuseini et al.(2016).

knife causes no pain. A number of scientists don't agree with this. Moreover, as John Webster (2005) has pointed out, a major (if not the) source of distress to an animal which has its throat slit is that it is aware it is in essence choking on its own blood. For this reason, religious slaughter is unsatisfactory and unacceptable on welfare grounds. But this is a political hot potato. Many think that human rights (ie right to behave according to what your religion tells you to do) trump any consideration of animal welfare. New Zealand banned kosher and halal slaughter (ie without stunning) in 2010. There was a ferocious outcry, particularly from the Jewish community. On this subject, I find myself disagreeing with Alex Bruce (it's rare). I think moral issues should be dealt with in a way which is not subject to special pleading. There is, I think, no difference between taking the view that religious slaughter is wrong, and taking the view that older men should not have sex with females below the age of sixteen. Some people in some cultures would disagree with the latter premise. But that is the law in Australia, and everyone should abide by it. The same can be said of non-stun slaughter according to religious ritual.

With her characteristic bluntness, Temple Grandin has said regarding abattoirs '...there are still problems when nobody is watching'.[483] Recent undercover footage of what goes on in Australian abattoirs has convincingly demonstrated that the law governing slaughter of animals in abattoirs is inadequate. This has been acknowledged by the New South Wales Food Authority, responding to revelations at Hawkesbury abattoir (in 2012), which has conducted a review of the adequacy of the core welfare provision (the abattoir code: AS4696:2997). It found that the animal welfare section of the code is 'inadequate by itself to assess compliance with animal welfare practices'. Instead, the Authority recommends compliance with the Australian Meat Industry Council 'Industry Animal Welfare Standards' for abattoirs (2nd edition, 2009). This latter set of standards is an audit-based procedure, reflecting the protocols designed by Professor Temple Grandin. This is a laudable step.

---

[483] Grandin (2013).

Even more importantly, there is a move to more rigorous monitoring and inspection, with closed circuit TV monitoring of all abattoirs. Unfortunately there is little sign of other jurisdictions adopting such an approach. Contrast this with the situation in the European Union, where monitoring of stun quality is mandatory.[484]

---

[484] Council Regulation (EC) No 1099/2009, on the protection of animals at the time of killing.

# Chapter 7    Live export

In my view, the number one animal welfare issue in Australia today is the live export of sheep, cattle, buffalo and goats for slaughter and breeding. The live export trade has been controversial since its inception in the 1970s. In the main, it is not popular with the public, yet farmers and their representatives clearly feel the need to defend it vigorously.

Commercially, live export is to animals what export of iron ore is to car manufacture. It's not so much dig it up and ship it out, but grow it up (to a certain extent), then ship out the jobs and the value-adding. With the touted expansion of live cattle exports to China,[485] pushed by (then) federal Agriculture Minister Barnaby Joyce's friend Gina Rinehart, a cynic might say we will soon be importing our own beef back from China. We shall see. In the meantime, Labor and Liberal-National politicians prostrate themselves before the false idol of live export, conveniently ignoring the obvious: the best way to export meat from Australia is to kill the animals in Australia and export the meat chilled or frozen. It is not good to cram animals into a ship, with barely enough room to lie down and to subject them to a long and risky journey, which will probably kill significant numbers of them, and cause serious distress and ill-health to many more. And that's just the live export journey; it goes without saying that the fate of the animals at the other end is a complete lottery, and likely to be pretty nasty. This is what every animal welfare expert and veterinary body would say. Yet today, live export has become the line in the sand; farmers across the board, and most politicians in both major parties continue to deceive the public regarding the animal cruelty inherent in live export. Live export just cannot be criticised in any way, such is the sensitivity of the farming lobby to this issue. The reason for this frantic defence of live export is, I think, that the setback suffered by the industry after the revelations of 2011, when animal welfare advocates could be said to have scored a

---

[485] It is claimed there will be up to one million head of cattle per year exported to China.

win, was too much for farmers and animal use industries to tolerate. Since that time, there has been an enormous backlash, which has served to further entrench the cruel practices of the live export trade.[486]

To me, live export is something Australians should be deeply ashamed of.

### Background[487]

Live export really began to grow with the export of end-of-life wool producing Merino sheep. In the 1970s, when the trade developed, the vast majority of exported sheep were castrated males, or wethers. These animals were essentially worthless. Western Australia was and remains the source of most live export sheep and Middle East countries remain the major market for sheep. The ships involved were mainly small converted oil tankers. As the trade picked up, some of the larger ships were able to carry up to 130,000 sheep. This trade peaked in about 1987, when 7.2 million sheep were exported to countries in the Middle East. The cattle trade developed later. It involved animals mainly from northern Australia (ie northern Western Australia and Queensland, and the Northern Territory). The meat from these *Bos Indicus* animals has traditionally not been attractive to the domestic market, which favours European *Bos taurus* breeds, such as Angus and Hereford. The predominant market for the cattle exported from northern Australia was and remains Indonesia. Export of cattle reached a peak of 1.3 million in 2014-15, with Indonesia taking about 750,000 of these animals.[488]

It is obvious that the motivation for farmers is a price premium for animals sold for live export. These higher prices are presumably offered in arrangements made directly between the exporters and the farmers. The corollary is that those seeking to buy animals for domestic slaughter

---

[486] Jones and Davies (2016).
[487] See Caulfield (2009), the website of Vets Against Live Export at www.vale.org.au, and Jones and Davies (2016) for more detailed background.
[488] ABARES (2016).

may not be able to make a profit buying animals at the price that the exporters offer. Thus, a serious and ongoing consequence of exporting animals live is the resultant closure of many Australian abattoirs, particularly in the north. This created a situation where many northern cattle producers became completely wedded to, and dependent on live export.

Live export from Australia has been heavily criticised on animal welfare grounds for many years. Even disregarding what happens to the animals in the importing countries, it is clear that the voyage itself presents significant animal welfare issues. To understand this, it is necessary to get an idea of what the live export process involves. Sheep and cattle can be subjected to very long journeys of up to 6 weeks, such as in the case of cattle transported to Russia. Extremes of temperature and humidity are often encountered when crossing tropical and equatorial regions *en route* to the northern hemisphere. On board ship, the animals are fed processed pelleted food. As most animals are reared on pasture, they must be acclimatised to this food before they are loaded onto the ship. This transition occurs in feedlots designated as 'registered premises' for pre-embarkation assembly of animals. In the case of sheep, transition to pelleted feed comes with its own particular problem. A significant minority will fail to eat the pellets, either in the registered premises, or on board the ship. They will starve to death on the voyage, or be so seriously weakened they will die from other causes, including disease or trauma. Other animals will succumb to infections, for example salmonellosis, while others will die of heat stress. Obviously a combination of all these factors can be lethal. In the case of heat stress, the limited space allocated to the animals makes things worse, as the sheep or cattle simply cannot dissipate the heat they generate. The average sheep gets just one third of a square metre of space, while the average cow gets about 1.25 square metres. This means in extreme conditions they just cook from the inside.[489] Those that do not die will nevertheless suffer considerably.[490]

In 1985, the Senate committee on animal welfare reported on the live sheep trade to the Middle East and said:

> *'if a decision were to be made on the future of the trade purely on animal welfare grounds, there is enough evidence to stop the trade...[which is] inimical to good animal welfare, and it is not in the interests of the animal to be transported to the Middle East for slaughter.'*

The Committee identified the urgent need for improvement of animal welfare in the live sheep trade, but said that whatever was done, there would still be significant stress, suffering and risk. The long-term solution, it said, was substitution of live export with export of refrigerated product. These conclusions were ignored.

After the 'roo in the stew' scandal of the 1980s, when so-called Australian beef exported to the USA was actually kangaroo meat, and the subsequent Woodward Royal Commission, the federal government enacted the *Export Control Act 1982*. This imposed certain requirements, such as notifications and so on, of exports of certain goods; the export of live animals was tacked on. In 1996 a government inquiry recommended reducing the regulatory burden on the meat industry (again including live animals in its consideration) by in effect introducing self-regulation. The basis for achieving this was the *Australian Meat and Live-stock Industry Act 1997* (the 'AMLI Act') and subordinate legislation. A key requirement of the AMLI Act was that an exporter of live animals had to have a licence (section 54). The self-regulation element was imposed by giving certain responsibilities to a private corporation, the Australian Livestock Export Corporation Limited, or 'LiveCorp'. Part of those responsibilities included the

---

[489] See Caulfield et al. (2014).
[490] Phillips (2016c).

development and administration of standards applying to the industry; live exporters were to be accredited against those standards, which were the *Australian Livestock Export Standards* (ALES). The standards were not developed with any animal welfare considerations in mind, rather they were 'practicable standards set by and for industry'.[491] The real consequence of this arrangement was that the industry, in the form of LiveCorp, decided whether or not an exporter should be licensed, and thereby had power to police the trade.

Things did not go well for the live export industry after this. There was a series of incidents involving the death of many thousands of animals on board ship, provoking a series of government inquiries and reports. But the government chose not to act.[492]

However, in August 2003 over 5,500 sheep died aboard the *Cormo Express* which was carrying 57,937 sheep to Saudi Arabia. The shipment was rejected by the Saudi authorities, who said sheep were infected with the disease scabby mouth. After more than 80 days at sea, the surviving animals were offloaded in Eritrea. The government responded to the huge outcry by instigating a review under Dr John Keniry. The Review was scathing in its assessment of self-regulation by the industry. It described the trade as 'uniquely and inherently risky'. It also drew the connection between live export and the wider Australian meat industry, saying 'the way it operates has implications for the industry as a whole.'

The major outcome was that LiveCorp had its responsibility for standard-setting taken away, although it has remained responsible for accrediting onboard stockmen. The government responded to other aspects of the report by announcing there would be nationally consistent standards focused on health and welfare. These key recommendations were not followed up. Instead, the *Australian Standards for the Export of Livestock* were created, not by independent animal welfare experts, but by government officers and industry

---

[491] See Caulfield (2008).
[492] See Caulfield (2008).

representatives. In many crucial respects these new standards were actually a rehash of the old standards. Space allowances for animals on ships, for example, were unchanged. Jones and Davies (2016) remark that those space allowances in essence reflect the number of animals which can be crammed into a given space, with no consideration given to whether or not they can lie down and get up again. While there was a requirement for a stockperson (who was an employee of the exporter) to be on every voyage, there was no requirement for a veterinarian to be on every ship. This was a requirement which could be imposed at the discretion of the Department, and the veterinarians who went on the ship when the Department did impose that condition were again not independent, but were employees of the exporter.

So what purported to be an exercise in removing self-regulation was in fact an exercise in imposing extra paperwork and ensuring that there was nobody on board live export ships who was independent of the exporter, and who could thereby report on animal welfare issues in an objective fashion. Since then, what happens on the ships remains hidden, with a conspiracy of silence and obfuscation involving the government, the exporters, the stockpersons and the on board veterinarians.

## The events of 2011[493]

In the years just prior to the Keniry Review, Lyn White of Animals Australia began to uncover evidence of cruelty to Australian animals in importing countries. Until then, the main concern had been with what happened to animals during the voyages; little was known about what went on once the animals arrived at their destinations. Most of Lyn's focus initially was on the Middle East, in countries such as Kuwait, Bahrain, Qatar, Oman and Egypt. As a result of what Lyn White found in Egypt, in 2006 the then federal minister for agriculture, Peter McGauran, suspended the export of live animals to that destination.

---

[493] Far and away the best source of information on this topic is *Backlash*, by Bidda Jones and Julian Davies (2016).

This was after he was presented with video footage of savage cruelty in the main Cairo abattoir (Basateen). At this time, the Department of Agriculture started entering into Memorandums of Understanding with several importing countries in an effort to gain control of issues relating to animal welfare. The main aim of these MOUs was to prevent another *Cormo Express* disaster by seeking to ensure that animals which were rejected by one country could go somewhere else. Even at the time those with knowledge of the industry thought these were nothing more than so much worthless paper, as they were without legal force.

Meanwhile the industry, in the shape of Meat and Livestock Australia and LiveCorp, with the active connivance of the government, was engaging in a propaganda campaign spruiking what they said were (taxpayer funded) improvements in animal welfare in importing countries, including Indonesia. In one sense this came back to bite them after the revelations of 2011.

In 2009, RSPCA Australia wrote to the industry and government requesting it be permitted to go to Southeast Asian countries to see what was happening to Australian animals there. That request was refused. However, what did happen was the industry put together a group, including two senior veterinary scientists (Professors Ivan Caple and Neville Gregory), which visited Indonesia to assess animal welfare in all parts of the live export supply chain in that country, which of course involved cattle. In 2010, the Department of Agriculture invited RSPCA Australia representatives, including Dr Bidda Jones (its Chief Scientist), to attend a meeting at which Professor Caple would present findings of the group's tour. Bidda Jones realised that, despite the oblique wording of the group's report, the descriptions of what went on in slaughterhouses in Indonesia raised many concerns. The report had, for example, described animal welfare as 'generally good', despite clear indications that there were huge problems with the slaughter process. As a result, Lyn White of Animals Australia went to Indonesia in early 2011, and witnessed dreadful cruelty inflicted on Australian cattle at Indonesian abattoirs. She was able to take video footage of what she saw. I remember vividly at the time receiving emails from Lyn each evening on her return from some of those places describing her shock and horror. Bear in mind this is a woman who had in her time seen quite revolting things done to animals, for example in Cairo's notorious Basateen abattoir. There is little point reiterating what she observed. Suffice to say it was nightmarish. To make things much, much worse, a lot of what was going on involved a so-called restraint box installed in many locations, over several years, by Meat and Livestock Australia and LiveCorp. This is in fact a device designed to 'cast' the animal; what that means in real terms is that cows are almost ejected from the box (with legs roped, by the way) to fall sideways onto a concrete platform, often crashing their heads onto it in the process.[494] Altogether a most violent and unpleasant process.

Bidda Jones analysed White's footage, using tried and tested scientific techniques. This was a critical part of presenting a completely objective story setting out the scale of this animal welfare disaster. The ABC's *Four Corners* not only decided to run with the footage, it went to Indonesian slaughter facilities to see for themselves what went on.

The response to the *Four Corners* programme was unprecedented. There were nearly a quarter of a million signatures on an online petition organised by GetUp! just one week after the episode.[495]

Part of the reaction included repeated statements by meat and farming industry representatives that what happened in Indonesia was unacceptable.[496] Such views ceased to be expressed not long after the dust had settled about cruelty, and the focus turned to the hard-done-by farmers.

---

[494] The Chief Veterinary Officer, Dr Mark Schipp, subsequently produced a report saying in effect that this device was unacceptable on welfare grounds.
[495] Pendergrast (2015); Jones and Davies (2016).
[496] Pendergrast (2015).

Ultimately, the government response was to suspend live exports for five weeks, to institute an independent inquiry,[497] and following that inquiry, to put in place a scheme – the Exporter Supply Assurance System, or ESCAS, which it claimed would prevent these things happening again. The essence of the system was to seek to ensure traceability of Australian animals. All cattle (not sheep) would be individually identified and exporters would have to provide evidence (in essence based on contracts with people further down the line in the importing country) that animals would stay within a closed supply chain system. Likewise, exporters would have to provide evidence that abattoirs would be run in compliance with relevant OIE recommendations.[498] Auditors, which would be appointed and paid for by the exporters, would provide reports as to the level of compliance or otherwise. One of the things neither the inquiry nor ESCAS included was a requirement for animals to be stunned prior to slaughter.

What was not predictable, however, was the vigorous and sustained campaign mounted by the industry and its sympathisers once the uproar about animal cruelty had subsided.

### The backlash

It would seem that the effect of the ban on the trade, in terms of exports lost, was that about 100,000 fewer animals were exported in the second half of 2011 compared to the same period in 2010. On the other side of the ledger, the government gave financial assistance of various sorts amounting to just under $35 million, as compensation; this has been

---

[497] There was also an inquiry by a Senate committee. This turned into an onslaught of unsubstantiated allegations against Lyn White and Bidda Jones, primarily driven by Senators Bill Heffernan and Chris Back. Professor Ivan Caple suggested that some of the recordings had been doctored. Chris Back alleged that Lyn White had bribed local people to engage in the cruelty depicted. Despite saying he had solid evidence, no such evidence ever materialised. In an ironic twist, Chris Back has recently been appointed to oversee development of new onboard welfare standards.

[498] The OIE is an international body which makes recommendations about animal welfare and health.

described by industry as 'a drop in the ocean';[499] to this day (that is, over six years later) the industry complains that the effect of the ban was catastrophic and still being felt. Personally, I find this hard to believe.

While the events of 2011 following the *Four Corners* programme on live export were unprecedented, it is notable that once the government and industry were seen to have dealt with the issue (by the introduction of the Export Supply Chain Assurance Scheme, ESCAS), those in favour of abolishing live export lost traction with the media. Indeed media coverage of the issue slumped.

Another real consequence of the Indonesian revelations is that the industry and those associated with it tightened up security, with the result that it has become impossible for outsiders to see what is actually going on within the 'supply chain'.

In 2013 the Coalition came to power in federal parliament and very soon made it clear that the emphasis had completely shifted away from animal welfare, to the suffering farmers who had been penalised by the live export suspension, painted as an over-reaction on the part of the previous Labor government. Part of Prime Minister Tony Abbott's vilification of the Gillard Labor government was that the live export suspension was an over-reaction. Unfortunately, Labor politicians such as Joel Fitzgibbon were very keen to chime in. In a rush to curry favour with the farming lobby, the cruelty was forgotten by both sides of politics. The new Minister for Agriculture, Barnaby Joyce, was vocal in his support for live exports, saying that he was focused on increasing returns for farmers, and supporting live export was part of that focus. Ethical considerations had disappeared, and once again the main consideration was that anything goes, providing it makes a dollar. Even with an exclusively economic focus, the obsession with short-term strategies and profits, at the expense of any long-term strategy for the

---

[499] See Jones and Davies (2016).

domestic meat processing industry, seems destined to create future problems.

## The current position

### The law

Rather than engage in a tedious blow by blow account of what is in the law,[500] I think it is best to start at the end, with a quote from the foremost current source on live export, which sums up where we are:

> 'The industry brags about having the best standards in the world, because our standards are more detailed and prescriptive than any other country that is willing to participate in this trade. But those standards still fall far short of providing a good environment, and ensuring a duty of care, for the livestock they are intended to protect. The imperative for an exporter is that enough animals reach the other end alive...'.[501]

So, regardless of what is written in the law, the outcome of live export is very bad welfare for a lot of animals. And what is written in the law guarantees that bad outcome, primarily because the relevant standards are so much weaker than those applied under Australian domestic animal welfare law and are in any case unenforced.

There are two major statutes and one other statute having a minor role governing live export. These are the *Australian Meat and Live-stock Act 1997* (Cth) ('AMLI Act'), the *Export Control Act 1982* (Cth) ('Export Act') and the *Navigation Act 2012* (Cth). The AMLI Act deals mostly with matters relating to the licensing of live export. Orders made under the Export Act (*Export Control (Animals) Order 2004* (Cth)) cover matters such as required notifications and permissions, including the Exporter Supply Chain Assurance System. These orders in essence deal with individual consignments (there can be more than one consignment,

---

[500] There is extensive detail in the relevant section of *Halsbury's Laws of Australia*, written by me, to be published in 2018.
[501] Jones and Davies (2016).

involving more than one exporter, on a single voyage). Each consignment must be notified to the Department, which must issue an export permit before the export can proceed.[502] The *Marine Orders Part 43 2006* (Cth) are made under the *Navigation Act 2012*, and concern matters relating to ship infrastructure etc. The Department of Agriculture and Water Resources is the lead agency concerning live export matters, administering the AMLI Act and the Export Act.

It is an offence to export 'livestock' (which is defined) unless the putative exporter holds a licence.[503] If certain events occur concerning the export licence holder, including a breach of the licence conditions, the Department Secretary *may* (not must) issue a 'show cause' notice, and after allowing response(s) to that, *may* ultimately take action against the exporter, including to suspend the licence.[504] What is crucial to note is that the Secretary (ie the Department) is under no obligation to take any action against an exporter, no matter how grievously the exporter breaks the law, or breaches export licence conditions.[505] What that means, given the very cosy relationship between the Department and the exporters, and the express support of the Minister for live export, is that the Department does nothing, no matter how egregious the breach of the law.

### Australian Standards for the Export of Livestock ('ASEL')

It is a condition of an export licence that the holder must comply with ASEL.[506] ASEL is a set of standards which are not put before parliament, but which are prepared by the government and industry. Intentional

---

[502] *Export Control (Animals) Order 2004* o1A.24(2) (notice of intention to export); o1A.01(2)(j) (export permit).
[503] *AMLI Act* s54(2); the Secretary must be satisfied of various matters before granting a licence. Those include that the applicant is of integrity, competent to hold the licence and of sound financial standing: AMLI Act s 54(1).
[504] The relevant provisions are in s23 of the AMLI Act.
[505] see *Animals' Angels e.V. v Secretary, Department of Agriculture* [2014] FCAFC 173.
[506] *Australian Meat and Live-stock Industry (Standards) Order 2005*. The relevant version of ASEL is version 2.3 (2011).

contravention of a licence condition (or contravening a condition recklessly) is a serious offence.[507]

One important condition of ASEL is that there must be inspections of animals at various stages in the preparation of animals for a voyage, and animals which are not fit (according to defined criteria) must be rejected. Given the cursory nature of much inspection, it is likely that many animals go on live export voyages which should not.

ASEL defines the minimum space requirements for the animals on the ship. These are minuscule; about one third of a square metre for the average sized sheep and 1.25 square metres for the average cow. These space provisions are inadequate and must inevitably contribute to many animal welfare problems, not least of which is heat stress.[508]

There is no requirement under ASEL that a veterinarian should accompany every live export voyage. This occurs at the discretion of the Department. Furthermore, when the Department makes it a condition of an approval, the exporter gets to choose the veterinarian, who is contracted by the exporter. Each live export ship must have on board at least one accredited stockperson (accredited by the industry body LiveCorp) who is contracted to the exporter, regardless of whether or not there is a veterinarian on board. A major responsibility of these persons is to provide reports to the Department, including daily reports (for voyages greater than 9 days) and an end of voyage report. These reports must include various observations relevant to animal welfare, including mortality.

A key requirement imposed on the stockperson (or veterinarian, if present) is to inform the Department if a 'notifiable incident' occurs. This is defined by ASEL to include (in essence) 2% mortality for sheep and goats, and (for voyages greater than 9 days) 1% for cattle and buffalo. Bear in mind, though, that these reports are made by employed

---

[507] AMLI Act s54(3).
[508] Caulfield et al. (2014).

agents of the exporter. There is no independent reporting, and it is hardly surprising, therefore, that some veterinarians who have spoken out have indicated that the true mortality figures are often under-reported. Although the Department is not required to do anything in response to these incidents, in practice the Department will carry out an investigation if the thresholds are exceeded. These thresholds for mortality reflect a very important difference between animal welfare standards in domestic Australian law, and the law governing live export. In all Australian jurisdictions it is an offence to be cruel to *an animal* (that is, a single animal). Cruelty can include not providing adequate food or water or otherwise causing animals harm. So cruelty which is well short of killing an animal as a consequence is a crime; the opposite is true of live export, where the practical outcome is that a high level of mortality is accepted as the norm. Suffering caused by the process is irrelevant. Reports of 'mortality investigations' are published, as are statements of actions taken against exporters. To my knowledge, since the changes in the law in 2004 after the *Cormo Express* incident, not one single exporter has had a licence taken away for excessive mortality, let alone cruelty. Reading the reports, it is evident that the Department is unprepared to take action, even though the whole process is bound to cause a high level of suffering for many animals. The most the Department ever does is say there must be greater space provision on the next voyage (usually 5% or 10%). There is no rationale to this; the only possible explanation is that it represents a *de facto* punishment for the exporter, who on a full ship, cannot carry as many animals. All of that is dependent, of course, on someone actually enforcing the space requirements. In my view this is unlikely.

### Exporter Supply Chain Assurance System ('ESCAS')

ESCAS applies to animals exported to be slaughtered fairly soon after arrival in destination countries, or to be fed in lots for a time, before slaughter. It does not apply to cattle exported for breeding purposes. This probably results in the exclusion of over 100,000 cattle per year from regulation under ESCAS.[509] As Jones and Davies (2016) point out, all an exporter has to do to avoid oversight is designate a cow as a breeder.

A key condition of approval of an ESCAS is that animals are slaughtered in compliance with the 'recommendations and standards' of section 7 in the Terrestrial Health Code of the World Animal Health Authority (the 'OIE'). This has often been touted as a plus point of ESCAS, along the lines that ESCAS requires compliance with 'world standards'. This is misleading. The OIE does not in fact publish standards. It makes recommendations. They are not intended to be best practice. Jones and Davies (2016) note that compromise between the OIE member countries at a variety of stages of development reduces the recommendations to the lowest common denominator. For example, section 7.5 of that Code ('Slaughter of Animals') allows slitting of an animal's throat without stunning. Worse, still, this section allows hobbling, casting or inversion of animals. These are exactly the techniques which were in use in Indonesia and were exposed in the ABC *Four Corners* programme in 2011.

There are suggestions that the ESCAS approach has achieved some improvement. For example, it is claimed by the industry that about 90 per cent of cattle exported to Indonesia are stunned before their throats are cut.[510] There is no way of independently verifying this.

Compliance with the conditions of an ESCAS is not routinely monitored by the Department of Agriculture and Water Resources. Responsibility for compliance is instead delegated to third party auditors, paid for by the exporters. Goodfellow (2015) points out that in the first year of its operation there were many reported breaches of ESCAS, many of which the Department found to be substantiated. Despite this, there were no

[509] In the year ended July 2017 118,000 breeder cattle were exported; Meat and Livestock Australia /LiveCorp *LiveLink July 2017*.
[510] Productivity Commission (2017).

sanctions other than to impose conditions on subsequent shipments.[511] As Goodfellow says, this is just a *de facto* tax, which the exporters accept as part of the cost of doing business.

RSPCA Australia, in a submission to the Productivity Commission, has seriously questioned the audit and approval process in ESCAS. It notes that the number of cattle exported to Vietnam increased by about 100 fold in the space of a couple of years (over 300,000 were shipped in 2015), and that 'there are now more Australian Government-approved abattoirs in Vietnam than there are abattoirs operating in Australia'. RSPCA Australia's view was that this was evidence of a 'rubber stamping' approach to audit and approval.

The most recent review of compliance with ESCAS covers the period 1 December 2016 to 28 February 2017,[512] during which time 519,000 relevant animals were exported to 14 markets.[513] Twelve investigations into non-compliance were completed during this time; the findings included 4 'critical' and 5 'major' incidents where there was non-compliance. Of all the reports which were investigated (ie 12), Animals Australia is listed as the complainant on 9 occasions. This is particularly interesting as, since the revelations of cruelty in 2011, it has been virtually impossible for non-industry personnel to gain access to slaughter facilities. So in other words, an independent charity, which has no rights of access, is acting as the main 'policeman' of the trade. However, it is probably fair to say that the presence of Animals Australia representatives in the importing countries may well be prompting exporters and others to 'self-report' breaches. What is clear from reviewing the summary report is that, no matter how bad the practices

---

[511] see also Productivity Commission (2017).

[512] www.agriculture.gov.au/export/controlled-goods/live-animals/livestock/regulatory-framework/compliance-investigations/investigations-regulatory-compliance/escas-reg-performance-rep-dec15-feb16

[513] Bahrain, China, Indonesia, Israel, Japan, Jordan, Kuwait, Malaysia, Oman, Philippines, Qatar, Turkey, United Arab Emirates and Vietnam.

observed, the Department does little more than slap the wrist of the exporters. The worst thing that happens is that facilities are 'suspended' from ESCAS approval; that presumably means the exporter just sends the animals elsewhere. The complaints made included observations of non-compliant slaughter in a Kuwaiti abattoir (which had previously been reported for non-compliance), sheep being tied up and dragged, and put in car boots, unapproved slaughter methods in Lebanon and Malaysia, and extensive 'leakage' of animals from what should be a closed supply chain.

The litany of ESCAS compliance failures is lengthy and repetitive. The only possible conclusion one can draw from these snapshots, made by a non-government agency under serious constraints, is that the system is not achieving what it set out to achieve. Moreover, no serious penalties are being applied.

Reflecting on what ESCAS means at its most basic, it is a requirement imposed on an exporter to have arrangements with third parties in importing countries to the satisfaction of the Department. But if those third parties do not keep to their side of the bargain with the exporter, how can the exporter possibly be the subject of action? It seems clear to me that if the Department took serious action against an exporter because of non-compliance with ESCAS conditions as a result of failures by, say, an abattoir operator in an importing country, it would be impossible for the Department to convince a court that the exporter was at fault. All the exporter has to do is have an appropriate arrangement in place which says it is going to satisfy ESCAS conditions. In other words, ESCAS is a system which is never going to work, because nobody can ever be held responsible in any serious sense.

There is an industry push for a co-regulation approach, based on the 'Livestock Global Assurance Program' currently being developed by the industry. It seems the gist of what the industry is aiming for is for the government to tick a box in effect exempting an exporter from separate auditing where an importing country has equivalent animal welfare standards. But this raises the obvious question of whether merely having laws and regulations in place is enough. Clearly it will not be enough if there is little or no enforcement.[514] The government has fallen into line with what the industry wants (which is tantamount to self-regulation) and has given $8.3 million to 'support the future implementation' of the program, whatever that means.

A primary motivation for all of this is to re-open the sheep trade to Saudi Arabia. Sheep have not been exported to Saudi Arabia from Australia since August 2012; it seems the Saudis were offended that anyone should think their facilities were not up to scratch and needed to be audited.

### The trade today

Surveys show that a slender majority of Australians would like to see live export banned. This does not paint the full picture. A survey of over 1000 people carried out by Utting Market Research in 2015 for Dr Heather Cambridge of Vets Against Live Export showed that a very large majority (84%) wanted independent veterinarians on board every live export ship, and a similarly large majority wanted standards equivalent to domestic Australian animal welfare law to apply throughout the live export chain. But the implication is that people are not aware that veterinarians on board ships are not independent, and the animal welfare standards applying to live export are substantially lower than domestic animal welfare law. I suggest that if domestic animal welfare standards were applied, and there was an independent vet on every voyage, the industry would be hard put to survive.

The Australian Veterinary Association has now changed its policy on live export.[515] It says that food animals should be slaughtered as close to the site of production as practicable and that there should be an

---

514 Productivity Commission (2017).
515 www.ava.com.au/policy/151-live-animal-export

independent veterinarian on every voyage. It also says that every step in the live export chain should be audited by independent auditors.

Meanwhile, the live export industry steadfastly maintains the position that 'animal welfare regulations' are too stringent, and reduce the competitiveness of the industry; thus importing countries can source animals from other sources where there are less demanding animal welfare requirements.[516] In other words, the live export industry (and presumably the farmers who service them) do not care one iota about animal welfare. It is important to bear this in mind for the next disaster to be revealed (as it surely will be), when we again will hear farmers and industry representatives, standing with a straight face, saying such cruelty is unacceptable – but we now know that the qualifier is 'providing we don't lose a single dollar'.

The scene today for live export is very different from the position a couple of years ago. The industry is struggling to find enough animals to fill orders, and more importantly, it is struggling to find importers who will buy animals at a price where they can make a profit, given the record prices being paid to Australian farmers for both sheep and cattle. It is continuing to export animals to volatile markets; when problems occur with one market (as is currently happening with Indonesia), they try and kick the can down the road by finding somewhere else to send the animals. And all the time Australian abattoirs are closing; the biggest domestic abattoir in Australia (Churchill, in Queensland) has announced its closure.[517] This is not a sensible business model. Nor is it good for the country. The obsession Australian governments have in maintaining the trade, for the extra few dollars it puts in some farmers' pockets, is penalising the rest of the country. Jobs and value adding by the meat

---

[516] www.abc.net.au/news/rural/2017-05-05/report-finds-welfare-rules-hinder-trade/8406764

[517] www.beefcentral.com/processing/churchill-abattoir-closure-leaves-woolworths-without-a-northern-beef-kill

processing sector is being steadily lost, while politicians blithely defend the economically and ethically indefensible.

The sources of animals exported live remains roughly the same. Many of the cattle which go into the live export trade – headed mostly for Southeast Asia, come from northern Australia. Most of the farms are on very marginal land, verging on desert. In most years there will be one muster at best. The animals are virtually feral and it seems that many of the animals which are mustered are not of the right weight or quality to go on a live export ship. During the dry season, there is almost nothing to eat. When I visited the Kimberley a couple of years back, I saw cattle which were extremely undernourished, seemingly surviving by eating bark from trees. There was no grass visible anywhere. But bearing this in mind, it is quite possible that the almost-feral animals living in this semi-desert may only be suitable for live export. This is because the country just does not sustain growing the animals up to slaughter weight, and there is a shortage (if not absence) of local slaughter facilities. If this is in fact the case, then governments need to grasp the nettle and acknowledge that growing animals in this entirely marginal country is bad for animal welfare and bad for the environment. Given there is no need to export meat by having it walk off a ship on four legs, this northern cattle trade in live animals should be substituted by boxed and frozen meat exports to the importing countries.

For sheep (which still come predominantly from Western Australia), it does seem as if the situation has changed quite drastically since the commencement of live sheep exports in the 1970s. The average weight of animals exported has fallen steadily since then, as the wool industry has diminished, and the animals available for live export are no longer the end of life wool-producing heavy wethers which has incidentally probably contributed to the steady reduction in overall mortality rates on voyages. Furthermore, the majority of Western Australian farms are mixed enterprises, engaging in crop production and also raising sheep or lambs.[518] The practical consequence of this is that live exporters are now competing directly with meat processors for the same sheep.

Over the years, supporters of live exports, primarily those who make money from the trade, have sought to distract attention from the inevitable cruelty associated with the trade by putting forward several justifications for continuing live export:

- *The live export industry is essential for Australian agriculture.*[519] Given it represents a small fraction of the total Australian animal industry, it is difficult to see how this can be so. Most farmers do not rely on live export for their income.
- *Because Australia exports live animals to countries where it seeks to improve animal welfare, then live export must continue otherwise there would not be a continuing animal welfare improvement in those countries.* As Bidda Jones and Julian Davies put it, 'again and again, breaches of standards reveal how little control or influence we have over our animals once they leave our shores'.[520] This is true, and in any case, a moment's reflection will reveal that people who are driven by profit would not for a moment be motivated by a consideration of animal welfare in an importing country.
- *Importing countries are not prepared to accept chilled or frozen meat.* The argument is that these countries lack the proper infrastructure to refrigerate meat, particularly where it has to be transported large distances. The other argument, thrown in for good measure, is that many of the importing countries have a tradition of meat being bought at so-called 'wet markets'. At the time of writing, it is apparent that both of these arguments are baseless. For example, the Indonesian market for Australian cattle is under severe stress because of competition from Indian

---

[518] ACIL Tasman (2009).
[519] see www.livecorp.com.au/about-us/introduction.
[520] Jones and Davies (2016).

frozen buffalo meat. This is meat, not live animals. This started coming into the Indonesian market in about June 2016. Since then, it has claimed roughly 20% of the total beef market in Greater Jakarta and is present in over 40 'wet markets' in Jakarta and elsewhere.[521] Record prices for Australian cattle have meant they are less able to compete effectively in the Indonesian market. This is evidenced by the recent announcement that Australia's largest live exporter, Wellards, will seek funds from shareholders by issuing 25 million shares in a bid to compensate for reduced income as a result of record high cattle prices.[522] The news from Wellards is they have made a loss of nearly $80 million in 2017.[523]

- *Live export, and the beef and sheep meat export markets, are separate markets.* In other words, animals exported live would not be able to go into the domestic and export meat processing chain; there would therefore be no competition in the ultimate export markets. As with all the other justifications, this has evaporated over the last couple of years. It is now clear that the live export of sheep and cattle, coupled with a reduction in the national cattle herd and sheep flock, is throttling the supply of animals for abattoirs in many parts of Australia. Several of those abattoirs have closed or are running truncated hours. Ross Ainsworth, writing on the excellent website *Beef Central*[524] illustrates this. In his report he includes a photograph of

---

[521] Beef Central 3 April 2017 'MLA surveys impact of Indian buffalo meat in Indonesia'. www.beefcentral.com/live-export/indonesia/mla-surveys-impact-of-indian-buffalo-meat-in-indonesia.

[522] ABC Rural 3 April 2017 'Livestock exporter Wellard turns to shareholders to raise funds as record high cattle prices put pressure on trade'. www.mobile.abc.net/news/2017-04-03/wellard-to-ask-shareholders-to-help-raise-$52-million/84108807?pfmred.

[523] www.abc.net.au/news/rural/2017-08-31/wellard-livestock-export-$77-million-loss/8859080.

[524] www.beefcentral.com/live-export/se-asia-report/se-asia-report-indonesian-importers-being-squeezed-from-all-sides/

products on their way to a wet market in Java, Indonesia. In the picture are two boxes of frozen Australian beef, a box of frozen Indian buffalo meat, and part of a cow carcase. How can the live export industry and indeed Australian famers and the government maintain the illusion that live export does not compete with Australian meat exports in the same market?

- *If we didn't do it, someone else would.* On this argument, any immoral, but profitable activity, would be justified.

The other justifications, which are really too silly to give space to, are set out and dealt with by Bidda Jones and Julian Davies in their book.[525] But however delusional this self-serving industry propaganda is, it has been swallowed by the politicians and probably (unfortunately) by a fair section of the public.

Regardless of the success of the propaganda, live export is currently struggling with economic realities. For example, the Indonesian government, seeking to grow its own cattle herd, has instituted a policy whereby importers of cattle must import one breeder animal for every five feeder (ie slaughter) animals. This has had the effect of reducing live cattle exports to that country.[526]

As of the end of 2017, the export of live cattle continues to decline, compared to the previous year's levels. The July 2017 statistics from Meat and Livestock Australia show a 24% drop in cattle exports compared to the previous year (just under 890,000). It is therefore likely that the value of cattle exports for 2017 will be considerably less than the value of almost $1.4 billion dollars for cattle exports in 2014-15 and about $1.6 billion for 2015-16. To put this into perspective, the value of

---

[525] Examples include that live export provides essential protein to poverty-striken people in importing countries, and that religious requirements demand live animals for meat.

[526] Meat and Livestock Australia 17 November 2016. 'Cattle exports slow amid Indonesian policy shift'. www.mla.com.au/prices-markets/market-news/cattle-exports-slow-amid-indonesian-policy-shift.

beef and veal exports for 2015-16 was about $8.3 billion. For Indonesia, imports of cattle from Australia declined from about 580,000 head for the year ending July 2016 to about 506,000 head for the year ending July 2017; 2016 saw record import by Indonesia of about 62 kilotonnes of beef from Australia.[527]

Live export of sheep has been decreasing steadily for the last ten years or so. 2.01 million sheep were exported in 2015; this was the second lowest number recorded since 1985. It appears that even fewer were exported in 2016 (about 1.9 million), and the figure for the year ending July 2017 is 1.7 million. In 2015-16 the value of live sheep exports was about $230 million;[528] The value of lamb and mutton exports for the same period was about $660 million.

I am firmly convinced that the voyage endured by animals exported live is unavoidably cruel. It is a fact that the mortality rate on a live export voyage, if applied throughout a herd or flock over a year, would result in the loss of over 25% of the animals.[529] Professor Clive Phillips estimates that the mortality rate for sheep on live export voyages is about 14 times higher than that for sheep on farms in Australia.[530] I am also convinced that the Department of Agriculture and Water Resources has no interest in ensuring that the legal requirements in relation to a live export voyage are complied with. In 2013 Dawn Lowe of Animals' Angels, myself and barrister Naomi Sharp commenced an action in the Federal Court against the Department. The essence of the action were allegations that the exporter concerned in a voyage of the MV *Hereford Express* in late 2008 had (amongst other things) told the onboard vet to leave the ship before the end of its journey (it had stopped in Singapore on the way to Malaysia), altered the vet's report to under-report the level of mortality of goats, did not comply with the requirement to

---

[527] Meat and Livestock Australia *Australian beef exports monthly trade summary March 2017*.

[528] *Livelink April 2017* Meat and Livestock Australia.

[529] see Jones and Davies (2016).

[530] Phillips (2016c),

supply the Department with daily voyage reports, did not comply with the requirement to give the Department an end of voyage report covering the entire voyage and did not comply with the requirement to have a stockperson on board at all times.[531] All of these allegations were brushed aside by the Department. Because of the way the relevant bit of the AMLI Act is written,[532] there is no obligation on the Department to take any action against an exporter which does not comply with the law. It is purely a choice for the Department. And that is what the Department did. It chose to do nothing.

Sheep continue to die from heat stress. In this regard, it is remarkable that the Department of Agriculture and Water Resources, when investigating live export incidents for sheep, refers to a 'heat stress threshold', which it says is the 'maximum ambient wet bulb temperature at which heat balance of the deep body temperature can be controlled'.[533] This temperature is said to be 30.5 degrees Celsius; no indication is given as to the derivation of this figure. This is literally unbelievable, as the laboratory data (re-) analysed and reported by Caulfield et al. (2014) clearly show that the core body temperature of sheep starts to rise at wet bulb temperatures in excess of about 26 or 27 degrees Celsius.[534] This is graphically illustrated by what happened in September 2013, when a voyage carrying sheep to the Middle East experienced wet bulb temperatures in excess of 27 degrees Celsius for about 12 days. Unsurprisingly, large numbers of animals died from heat stress. Out of 44,713 sheep loaded in Adelaide, 3,256 died. Most of the animals died over a day or two when wet bulb temperatures peaked at

---

[531] *Animals' Angels e.V. v Secretary, Department of Agriculture* [2014] FCA 398. The appeal in *Animals' Angels e.V. v Secretary, Department of Agriculture* [2014] FCAFC 173, conducted by Naomi Sharp and Dr Jeremy Kirk SC, with Kiera Peacock of Marque Lawyers as solicitor, failed.
[532] see section 23(1) *Australian Meat and Live-stock Industry Act 1997* (Cth).
[533] see for example the investigation report at
www.agriculture.gov.au/export/controlled-goods/live-
animals/livestock/regulatory-framework/compliance-
investigations/investigations-mortalities/report-46.
[534] see Phillips (2016c)

around 34 to 35 degrees Celsius. This in itself indicates the nonsensical nature of the criteria applied by the Department, as despite this dreadful mortality, the temperatures never exceeded the 'mortality limit' of 35.5 degrees Celsius which the Department adheres to. This report also illustrates the classical response of the Department to a high mortality incident – the next voyage, in November, gave an additional 10% space to the animals. In other words, having had all these animals die of heat stress, the response was to change conditions for a voyage in the northern winter, when of course there would be very little likelihood of encountering such extremes of temperature and humidity. No other action was taken against the exporter. This confirms a longstanding impression, that the response which the Department always has, which has the effect (for a full shipload) of restricting the number of animals an exporter can carry, and thereby reducing its profit, is in effect a *de facto* penalty. It appears likely that there was a repeat performance in July 2016, when another sheep shipment to the Middle East (with 69,322 animals) had 3,027 deaths.[535] According to a record of actions taken by the Department,[536] once again heat stress was responsible for killing the animals. Unremarkably, the Department's response was to reduce the stocking density for the next consignment of that vessel. There is another response in that record of actions which illustrates the bizarre nature of regulation of this trade. It notes that 'heat stress...was a result of extreme humidity...'. It then goes on to say the Department required the exporter, for the next consignment, to load 'industrial fans to assist with ventilation'. This is completely weird, as if ambient temperatures and humidity were high enough for there to be heat stress, then no amount of ventilation will allow the animals to keep their body temperatures in a safe range. This

---

[535] See the relevant parliamentary report at
www.agriculture.gov.au/export/controlled-goods/live-animals/live-animal-export-statistics/report-to-parliament.
[536] www.agriculture.gov.au/export/controlled-goods/live-animals/livestock/regulatory-framework/compliance-investigations/investigations-mortalities/actions-delegate-jultodec2016

is because evaporative heat loss, which is crucial to avoid heat stress, will only be effective when humidity is low enough to allow evaporation.[537] Passive ventilation will never do this in high humidity conditions; only active cooling will work. Vets Against Live Export applied under Freedom of Information legislation for the various reports made by the onboard veterinarian in relation to this voyage. These revealed that there was extra space provided for the animals, which did not relieve the heat stress and resultant mortality; of course this also shows what we already know, which is that the mandated space allowances are grossly inadequate to prevent heat stress. Moreover, the data recorded showed that the surviving sheep gained weight. The implication here is that weight gain *per se* is not an indicator of good welfare, contrary to the sorts of statements frequently made by the industry and its supporters – clearly the dead sheep did not gain weight.[538]

There was a stunning failure of the ESCAS system in August 2012, when 20,000 sheep were rejected by Bahraini authorities on the grounds there were animals in the shipment with scabby mouth. There was a Memorandum of Understanding in place between Australia and Bahrain which should have guaranteed the sheep were put into quarantine, but this was ignored – as I have said earlier, these documents are, in a legal sense, worthless. The exporter, Wellards, had realised there were problems brewing and had obtained an import permit from Pakistan, as an alternative destination, even before the rejection by Bahrain. Pakistan had not previously been approved as a destination under the ESCAS system, but clearly the paperwork must have been shuffled pretty quickly by the Department to allow the animals to go there. Unfortunately neither the exporter nor the Department told the Pakistani authorities the animals had been rejected by Bahrain on the grounds there was disease. The facility the animals went to was not

---

[537] Caulfield et al. (2014).
[538] www.vale.org.au/uploads/1/0/4/3/10438895/ vale_press_release_170803.pdf.

even approved by the Pakistani authorities as a quarantine facility. The Pakistanis reacted by brutally slaughtering over 20,000 animals in the most horrendous fashion. All of this was reported by Four Corners as *Another Bloody Business*.[539] But this isn't the end of the affair. Part of what emerged about these events has formed the basis of charges laid against Garry Robinson, an export manager for Wellards. He was accused of two counts of dishonestly influencing a Commonwealth public official and one count of using a false Commonwealth document to obtain gain.[540] A document reported on by the ABC was allegedly said by Mr Robinson to have been described as having 'magic' done to it. The ABC has said that the documents used to gain permission to land the sheep in Pakistan 'appear to have been falsified'. Copies of some very interesting documents, including one seeming to relate to manipulation of mortality numbers, can be seen on the ABC website.[541] It appears that in January 2018 Mr Robinson pleaded guilty to one charge of dishonestly influencing a Commonwealth public official. The other two charges have been dropped.

Other documented failures of the ESCAS system, which have been steadfastly ignored by the government, are detailed in Jones and Davies (2016).

For many years outsiders were ignorant of conditions on board live export vessels. Veterinarians and stockpersons on board the ships are employed by the exporters and it is hardly surprising that they are reluctant to speak out about those conditions. When they do, they are blackballed by the industry. This was the case with the unique revelations by live export veterinarian Dr Lynn Simpson, whose continued employment in the live export section of the Department of Agriculture and Water Resources was deemed to be impossible when

---

[539] For details see the Vets Against Live Exports website at www.vale.org.au/media.html.
[540] Nick Butterly 'Ex-sheep ship boss charged' *The West Australian* 22 October 2016.
[541] www.abc.net.au/7.30/content/2014/s3985413.htm

the live export industry said they would no longer work with her. This was because the Department, contrary to her wishes, had made public a confidential submission by her to an inquiry into ASEL. That submission expressed the view, never expressed before by a veterinarian with shipboard experience, that stocking densities were too high, that 'acceptable' mortality rates were too high, that many animals were loaded which exceeded the rejection criteria (including loading animals which were far too heavy) and there was inadequate bedding. There was a particular concern about hard flooring causing serious foot and leg problems in cattle, often requiring them to be killed. Simpson's submission contained many photographic records, never before seen. Some of these images were very shocking, particularly those of cattle covered in faeces. There were many other issues raised in Simpsons' submission, but clearly this telling of the truth was not what the industry or the Department wanted.

In an amazing show of bravery, Simpson has continued her revelations with posts on the shipping industry website 'Splash 24/7'.[542] These often confirm what we have long suspected, for example that in fully loaded ships it is almost impossible to properly observe and monitor the health status of individual sheep in pens on ships, that many sheep and cattle still suffer and die from disease, that animals are often covered with faeces, and so on and so on.

Given this, and given what we now know in some detail about what goes on overseas, nobody can deny (and that includes the government) that this trade is an abomination which cannot be justified.

---

[542] www.splash247.com/tag/dr-lynn-simpson/

## Appendix 7    The law relating to live export

*Declarations etc*

Persons concerned with the live export process are required by the relevant law to make declarations, provide information or make returns to the Secretary of the Department of Agriculture and Water Resources; it is an offence to do any of those things knowing they are false or misleading in a material particular or recklessly as to whether they are false or misleading in a material particular. [543]

*Permissions for each voyage*

Export is prohibited unless various things are done, including:

- there is an approved Exporter Supply Chain Assurance Scheme (ESCAS);
- the Department has received from the exporter and approved a notice of intention to export for the export ;
- the livestock are held before export and assembled for export in registered premises (a feedlot);
- there is an approved arrangement for the exporter;
- the livestock have been prepared in accordance with the approved arrangement and any applicable conditions on that approval;
- the exporter has obtained an export permit for the export;
- the livestock are exported to the place and by the means specified in the export permit;
- the exporter complies with the approved arrangement, the approved ESCAS and any conditions, and
- the exporter complies with any condition of the export permit.

## ASEL

ASEL is made up of 6 standards, dealing with sourcing and on-farm preparation, land transport, livestock in registered premises (feedlots), vessel preparation and loading, onboard management and air transport.

## Approved arrangement

When the law was changed in 2004, part of the system put in place required an exporter to submit a 'consignment risk management plan' for each shipment. This requirement

---

[543] See, for example, *Australian Meat and Live-stock Industry Act 1997* s 11(3) (application for licence); *Export Control (Animals) Order 2004* ss 1A.02 (application for approval of arrangements for preparation of live-stock),1A.09 (application for proposed variation of approved arrangement), 1A.19 (application for approval of exporter supply chain assurance system), 1A.24 (notice of intention to export),1A.29 (application for export permit and health certificate), 2.04 (application for registration of premises for holding and assembling livestock), 4A.04(2) (application by veterinarian for accreditation), 4A.15 (report on export voyage to Secretary of Department of Agriculture and Water Resources by accredited veterinarian). *Australian Meat and Live-stock Industry Act 1997* s 55(1); *Australian Meat and Live-stock Industry Act 1997* s 55(2).

has now been removed. Instead, exporters can apply for an 'approved arrangement' with the Department, which is in essence a description of how the exporter will comply with all the various requirements (including requirements of the importing country: *Export Control (Animals) Order 2004* o1A.02(1)(a).

# Chapter 8    Use of animals in teaching and research[544]

In my view, the use of animals in biological research has contributed much to human knowledge and wellbeing.[545] The use of the past tense is important, as I am not convinced that in the future, advances in biomedical sciences will require animal research. We may have even arrived where we are today without animal experiments, but that is truly imponderable. Much of what was done and is still being done is at the high end of the cruelty scale, and thus there is still great public concern about the use of animals in science. A 2013 poll commissioned by Humane Research Australia found that 64% of those surveyed did not believe humans have a right to experiment on animals. A majority (56%) did not believe results obtained in animals were relevant to humans. There was great support for providing significant funds to seek alternatives to animal experiments (over 70%).[546] The real question, of course, is whether enough is enough. We cannot undo the past, but do we need more scientific research using animals in the future?

The use of animals in research stirs up more heated emotions than other activities which exploit animals, including breeding and killing them to eat. Katrina Sharman has described the scientific use of animals as 'one of the hardest issues to write about', and has said that 'the horrors that take place behind laboratory doors in the name of science, education and progress' raise 'some of the most difficult and confronting questions'.[547] Alex Bruce (2012) has said 'the use of animals for excruciatingly painful and frequently fatal scientific experiments raises some of the most difficult issues in contemporary society'. This latter statement does not address the question of how much of the

---

[544] I am very grateful to Dr Donald Straughan OBE, formerly (*inter alia*) UK Home Office Inspector (with responsibility for monitoring animal experiments), for his comments on this section.

[545] see Webster (2005).

[546] see www.theconversation.com/why-australia-needs-to-catch-up-on-animal-research-transparency-27169.

[547] Sharman (2006).

research in Australia does fall into that category of 'excruciatingly painful and frequently fatal', and what the purpose of that research was. Personally, I see little distinction in moral terms between subjecting an animal to serious surgical mutilations, such as having its testicles removed without the benefit of anaesthesia, or imprisoning it in a tiny cage for the rest of its life (I'm thinking of intensive pig farming or battery chicken cages), and the high impact research experiments Alex Bruce has referred to. So if one is justifiable, why not the other? (of course, I seek to justify neither, personally).

Images of vivisection have in the past provoked violent actions by a minority directed against scientists. I have a concern that some of this extreme emotion directed at scientists who use animals is based to some extent on ignorance of what actually goes on. The tendency is to assume that where an animal is used, pain is caused. This is not necessarily so. However, the scientists do not help themselves by failing to be transparent and hiding behind propaganda, rather than dealing honestly with questions and issues.

At present, society is prepared to allow animals to be used in science. This is despite opinion polls showing that a majority of people do not want animals to be used in scientific research. Regardless, politicians do not want to engage in this issue, beyond taking minor action, such as talking about stopping animal use in cosmetic testing. As there is no political appetite for banning animal use in science, it nevertheless needs to be regulated in order to ensure there is not (unjustifiable) cruelty and wastage of animal lives. The question, of course, is who decides what is unjustifiable and on what basis. As with all other types of animal exploitation, what one person will regard as completely unacceptable will be regarded by another as completely justifiable.

The section in this Chapter on legislation will reflect on how 'acceptability' of a particular procedure or experiment is achieved in Australian law. The code governing scientific research and teaching use of animals in this country, developed by the National Health and

Medical Research Council, is, I think, theoretically completely adequate for the task of saying what can and can't be done, how animals should be kept, and so on. However, the key section concerning monitoring and enforcement is a failure, embracing the usual situation of self-regulation. Thus, the Code is a worthy collection of words, designed to maintain the *status quo*.

## History

*'I never have seen, nor ever can see, any objection to the putting of dogs and other inferior animals to pain, in the way of medical experiment, when that experiment has a determinate object, beneficial to mankind, accompanied with a fair prospect of the accomplishment of it...To my apprehension, every act by which, without prospect of preponderant good, pain is knowingly and willingly produced in any being whatsoever, is an act of cruelty'.*

So said Jeremy Bentham, one of the early heroes of animal protection, in a letter to *The Morning Chronicle* in 1825.

Animals were certainly being used in scientific experiments at the time of Descartes – that is in the first half of the seventeenth century. Peter Singer in *Animal Liberation* gives descriptions of scientific experiments of the time, where horrendous cruelty was ignored by virtue of the then-prevailing Cartesian view of animals as soulless machines.

During the 19th century, in parallel with concern about welfare of domestic and farmed animals, there was a growing outcry about vivisection. The word 'vivisection' means carrying out experiments (usually expressed as 'operations') on living animals (conscious and unconscious). However, one needs to be clear what 'vivisection' was at the time, in practical terms. Fundamentally, it was carrying out procedures of some kind or other on living and <u>conscious</u> animals, without anaesthetic. The inevitable consequence of vivisection was dreadful pain and suffering.[548]

Mike Radford (2001) writes that, compared with continental Europe, vivisection was not much in evidence in the UK until the 1860s. This was the point where serious campaigning against vivisection commenced. As well as many famous figures of the day, the Queen herself expressed concern about the practice. In 1874 the RSPCA proposed that experiments on living animals should be prohibited, except under licence. The scientists fought back with the establishment of the Physiological Society, which was the first of its kind in the world.[549] The government appointed a Royal Commission to look into the matter. In Radford's view, evidence given by several of the proponents of vivisection was in fact damning to their cause, including as it did statements to the effect that they would not use anaesthesia except where it was convenient (for them) and had no regard for an animal's suffering. The 1873 *Handbook for the Physiological Laboratory*, produced by Sanderson of University College London, compounded the problem, making virtually no reference to the need for anaesthesia. Sanderson and the other authors of the book were put in serious difficulties under questioning by the Commission. Klein, of St Bartholomew's Hospital, came across as particularly arrogant and callous.[550] There was, however, an intriguing undertone of vile foreign practices being unacceptable in England (Klein was German).

Following the Commission's report, Parliament enacted the 1876 *Cruelty to Animals Act*. This made it an offence to carry out experiments calculated to cause pain, with the proviso that such experiments were allowed where the end was in advancing physiological knowledge, saving or prolonging life or alleviating suffering. A licensing system, administered by the Home Office, was put in place. The 1876 Act

---

[548] Richards (1986).
[549] Richards (1986).
[550] Richards (1986).

remained as the framework regulating scientific experiments in the UK until as recently as 1986. The Physiological Society went from strength to strength, shaking off the Continental roots of physiology and establishing the discipline as a highly-regarded branch of biological and medical science.

At this point it should be noted that the practical outcome, by the end of the nineteenth century, was that the law (and practice) had changed things so that, while 'vivisection' was still allowed (that is, experiments on living animals), causing pain was heavily regulated. This meant that the majority of seriously invasive experiments on animals were no longer on conscious animals, but on anaesthetised animals. This is a crucial distinction. In fact, anaesthetic agents had been available in the 1840s.

As the twentieth century progressed, with great technological advances, the physiologists and medical scientists had in essence won the battle which had been started and fought in the previous century. The use of animals in scientific experiments proceeded almost without question, and as more discoveries were made, the pharmaceutical industry flourished. After the Second World War, there were major and rapid advances, with drugs such as antibiotics, analgesics, anti-convulsants, anti-inflammatories and drugs for the treatment of conditions as diverse as depression, schizophrenia, Parkinsonism, high blood pressure, duodenal ulcers and asthma becoming available in increasing number and variety. Discoveries in basic biology also continued apace, with emerging understanding of cellular biochemical processes, neuronal function and other key areas. Of particular importance was the application of the discovery of the structure of DNA and how proteins were encoded and made in cells to the elucidation of the roles of genes. The ability to isolate and modify those gene sequences and then transfer them to cells and whole organisms resulted in the entire new discipline of molecular biology.

Until the mid-1980s I think it can safely be said that the majority of scientific research on animals was conducted by people who rarely asked moral questions about what they were doing; science was free of ethical considerations.[551] Scientists were able to suspend 'normal' sensibilities.[552] I am not saying that these people were egregiously cruel, just that they did what they did without really thinking too deeply about it, much like a farmer might deal with an animal. At the time, things were made worse by the risk of violent attacks against scientists using animals. This promoted a culture of self-justification and secrecy. Even though scientists were aware that they were inflicting pain on animals, it rarely occurred to them (or veterinarians) that it was possible and desirable to alleviate the pain. That much has changed today.[553] Veterinary surgeons will now routinely give animals analgesics after they have had surgery, and scientists must take into account whether they can relieve pain without frustrating the objects of their experiments.

People often refer to the work of Russell and Burch (1959) in setting out a working scheme for reducing the number of animals used in experiments. The Russell and Burch principles are referred to as the 'three Rs', being 'replacement, reduction and refinement':

- *Replacement*: is it possible to achieve the scientific objectives without using live animals?
- *Reduction*: if replacement is not possible, what is the least number of animals necessary to achieve the scientific objective? This requires statistical analysis of the numbers necessary to test the scientific hypothesis under consideration. Using too few animals will mean all the animals have been wasted, because the results are worthless. Using too many means the extra animals' lives are wasted.

---

[551] see Rollin (2007).
[552] see Richards (1986).
[553] see Rollin (2016).

- *Refinement*: Better design of experiments, or use of better techniques, can reduce the amount of harm that is inflicted, or the number of animals which have to be used.

As with the provision of pain relief, it has taken many years for the '3Rs' concept to filter through to mainstream scientific thinking.

As I have said, I believe that experiments on living animals have generated great and useful knowledge of the functioning and physiology of the human body. This in turn led to advances in surgery and therapeutics. Even so, it is intriguing to speculate what might have been if experiments on animals had stopped, say in the nineteenth century. Would biological and medical science have been held back, or would it have been forced to move more quickly to non-animal experiments in order to make progress? But animal experiments continued, and the use of animals contributed to the development of a huge repository of knowledge. That is not to say, of course, that their continued use is justified. In my heretical view, *almost* the opposite is true today. At least, there is a need to look with a very jaundiced eye at modern use of animals for science.

## Animal use in science today
There are three possible positions regarding animal use in research:

- complete abolition;
- only certain types of experiments should be allowed, under certain circumstances (particularly where there is a high likelihood of benefit);
- all experiments should be allowed, if researchers think they are useful.[554]

---

[554] Gross and Tolba (2015).

The first position is one you would expect of animal rights activists, while the second is probably the one which would be supported by most members of the public. The last is historical.

Research in Australia which uses animals is concentrated in universities, research institutions, government facilities (such as CSIRO) and independent laboratories which do testing on behalf of others. Animals are also used for teaching purposes.

It is very important to note that research using animals is part of a competitive and high pressure industry, primarily centred on universities. Scientific research has become increasingly corporatised, as universities behave less as educational institutions and more as businesses. This must be borne steadily in mind when one considers the justifications put forward for using animals and the claims that such research is beneficial. The employers (ie the universities) are more and more using 'metrics' of scientists' performance to decide on their advancement or continued employment. One such metric is the number of their publications (preferably in highly-ranked journals) – scientists must 'publish or perish'.[555] This practice has been said to have led to an increase in the amount of trivial, false and unreproducible scientific results.[556] Scientists are strongly motivated to keep using animals and make claims of future benefit, simply because of the pressure they are under.[557] It has been said 'by accepting the *status quo*, a researcher can avoid dealing with the intrinsic ambiguity, the unknown unknowns of biology and instead take refuge in a self-perpetuating safe harbor of delusional certainty that requires very little in the way of brain power'.[558] This applies even more so where use of animals is concerned. Biomedical research is a not insignificant business in Australia, and it is reasonable to suppose that much of it involves use of animals. This statement of the slightly obvious means that a lot of

---

[555] Jarvis and Williams (2016).
[556] Bowne and Casadevall (2015); Jarvis and Williams (2016).
[557] Lazebnik (2015).
[558] Mullane and Williams (2015).

people depend for their employment and their careers on this research continuing. There is therefore a significant vested interest in allowing this research. As will be seen, the final judgments on whether research with animals proceeds are made by the scientists themselves. This creates obvious problems.[559]

The main organisation in Australia which funds research using animals is the National Health and Medical Research Council (NHMRC). The total research budget of the NHMRC in 2015-16 was nearly $900 million.[560] It is not clear how much of that figure involves animal use. Helen Marston of Humane Research Australia has advised that her understanding, based on what she has been told by the NHMRC, is that perhaps about 35% of the money spent goes on research involving animals. So this amounts to about $300 million each year from the NHMRC alone. Of the money which goes to universities, figures up to 2009 indicate that up to 64% was for 'basic research'; one might assume a significant portion of that would involve animals.[561] So there is a significant amount of public money spent on scientific research using animals. This is another reason why the justification for that research must be seriously scrutinised.

There is little on the NHMRC website which indicates how the organisation, in considering grant applications, deals with proposals to use animals in research projects. The 'Advice and Instructions to Applicants' makes no reference of any significance to considerations involving animals use. The NHMRC Funding Rules require that researchers funded by NHMRC adhere to the requirements of the *Australian Code for the Responsible Conduct of Research*, which in turn requires that research using animals is in compliance with the NHMRC *Code of Practice for the Care and Use of Animals for Scientific Purposes* (see below). Likewise, researchers are required to make a statement that they are familiar with that Code and will comply with it. The

---

[559] Rollin (2016).
[560] National Health and Medical Research Council Annual Report 2015.
[561] see www.nhmrc.gov.au/grants-funding'research-funding-statistics-and-data

guidelines for peer review of grant applications on the NHMRC website make no mention of the need for reviewers to consider whether there are non-animal alternatives. This does seem to me to be a significant omission. Nevertheless, Helen Marston of Humane Research Australia thinks, based on her information, that grants will often be awarded by the NHMRC subject to approval by an Animal Ethics Committee, of which more below. So it does appear as if the responsibility for checking animal use is justified ultimately devolves to these Committees. Moreover, if the grant is awarded depending on an animal ethics committee approving the protocols, then it would appear that the committees may be under pressure to let things go forward once the money is in place. This is not satisfactory.

Humane Research Australia does a tremendous job of collecting statistics recording animal use in science around Australia.[562] That in itself is a telling statement. There is no central government repository showing how many animals are used and what they are used for. Humane Research Australia calculates that the total number of animals used in Australia in 2015 was just over 10 million.[563] This number sounds very large. The problem is that it is almost impossible to find out how many experiments involving serious damaging interventions were done on which species. For example, when scientists count in animals in the wild which they have observed, they become recorded in the statistics. So in 2015, New South Wales counted over 4 million native animals which had been observed in environmental studies.

There is confusion about what is involved in use of animals for research. The predominant view is that where experiments are done to benefit humanity, then this is because of 'an interest in avoiding the pain and suffering associated with untreatable diseases and medical

---

[562] www.humaneresearch.org.au/statistics/
[563] At the time of writing there were no specific figures for 2015 from Queensland, South Australia, Western Australia, ACT and Northern Territory. Extrapolations have been made from figures for earlier years.

problems'.[564] Indeed this may well be what the average member of the public (and perhaps authors of animal law textbooks) believes. But so far as Australia is concerned, this logic does not *directly* apply. This is because there is very little drug discovery research using animals done in Australia. By that, I mean the large scale testing of many chemical compounds, followed by toxicological and pharmacokinetic studies, then clinical trials, formulating a product, and then licensing it for sale (note I do not refer to the *clinical* tests, which are usually done in hospitals, on patients, and probably do go on in Australia). This is not a trivial enterprise these days. Drug discovery, development and licensing is the province of the pharmaceutical industry, which has a negligible pre-clinical research presence in this country. Companies are based in the USA (eg Merck Sharp & Dohme, Eli Lilly, Bristol-Myers Squibb, Pfizer), the UK (GlaxoSmithKline), Europe (AstraZeneca, Aventis, Boehringer Ingelheim, Novartis, Bayer, Roche) and Japan (Eisai, Takeda).[565]

There are uses of animals other than drug discovery in the pharmaceutical industry, or assessment of toxicity. One important such use is 'basic research'. This is curiosity-driven; it is research into fundamental mechanisms of how biological systems work, although it can have an ultimate therapeutic or beneficial goal. Although there is much basic biological research in Australia, it is not clear how much of it involves animals. For example, much of the work which can be said to be justified because it aims to 'cure cancer' will involve very basic studies of the function of cells, usually in or from animals. This is because, at its simplest, 'cancer' is the result of normal differentiated, non-dividing cells turning into cells which multiply in an uncontrollable way. So obviously the study of why cells lose this inhibition on growth

---

[564] Bruce (2012).
[565] see the website of the International Federation of Pharmaceutical Manufacturers and Associations: www.ifpma.org.

and division is relevant. But completely basic research may only have a tenuous link to human or animal disease or health.

The New South Wales Animal Research Review Panel (see Appendix 8) does provide some more detailed information about which animals are used for which purposes.[566] For example in 2015 about 20,000 laboratory mammals (so mainly rats and mice, with some guinea pigs and a much smaller number of rabbits) were killed for 'basic research' – defined as to increase the basic understanding of the structure, function and behaviour of animals and processes involved in physiology, biochemistry and pathology.

Moreover, both goal-oriented or basic research can involve whole animals (for example psychological experiments, say on memory function), or it can even involve single cells, or molecules extracted from animal tissues. Most biochemical work is in the latter category. Where whole animals are involved, interventions can be severe. This is the sort of thing people imagine when they hear the word 'vivisection'. The worst and best known examples involve surgical operations where the animal recovers consciousness after the operation. The most extreme of such procedures may, for example, involve ablation of a particular brain area to study its function. This is what I mean when I say it is to some extent misguided to condemn all use of animals in scientific experiments. If people are prepared to kill animals for food, then presumably they will not object to killing animals (humanely – whatever that may mean) for scientific purposes. I would have thought the greatest likelihood is that the average person would object to severe procedures, where there is pain and suffering. So it is critical to know how many such procedures there are.

The New South Wales data[567] gives information about serious procedures, justified as 'basic research', which were carried out using animals in 2015. These include major surgery (under anaesthetic) with

---

[566] Animal Research Review Panel (2017) Annual Report 2015-16.
[567] Animal Research Review Panel (2017) Annual Report 2015-16.

recovery, death as an endpoint of the procedure and 'major physiological challenge'. This latter procedure type involves the animal being conscious throughout, and there is 'interference with physiological or psychological processes' which causes a 'moderate or large degree of pain and / or distress that is not quickly or effectively alleviated'. In 2015, there were just under 14,000 such procedures, which again involved mostly rats and mice, but with a small number of rabbits, pigs and sheep. Where the justification was 'human or animal health or welfare', there were about 30,000 rats and mice involved, a total of just under 1,000 cattle or sheep, and relatively small number of dogs, cats, horses and pigs. For 'regulatory product testing', about 14,000 mice and 2,000 guinea pigs were used. It is clear from the report that most of these latter animals were involved in 'lethality testing'. Many of these tests are said to be required by regulatory authorities. This illustrates how regulatory authorities are still wedded to the use of what is outdated and unjustifiable technology. In my view, these are the procedures which should be very carefully scrutinised as to their justification.

It is important to realise that basic research almost always formed the foundation on which subsequent discoveries were made. To illustrate this, I think it is helpful to consider a well known example concerning asthma treatments. Asthmatics will probably use an inhaler to relieve the symptoms of the disease. All of these 'relievers' contain a drug of the class known as 'adrenergic beta$_2$ receptor agonists'. The first major drug of this class was Glaxo's salbutamol (Ventolin).[568] The development of this drug would not have occurred without basic pharmacological research which defined the subtypes of receptors involved.[569] At the

---

[568] Although it was not the first. That was the drug terbutaline, produced by Swedish company Astra in 1966.

[569] Receptors are protein molecules, usually on the surface of cells (muscle cells, nerve cells, gland cells, etc), which recognise signals from outside, for example from hormones, such as adrenaline, or neurotransmitter chemicals released from nerves, and in response to those signals, produce a response in the cell containing the receptors. An example is the nicotinic acetylcholine

start of the 20th century, Abel isolated the hormone adrenaline. Sir Henry Dale's work in the early part of the 20th century demonstrated that adrenaline had two major different actions, one of which could be blocked by the substance ergotoxin (from a fungus which grows on plants such as rye). The effect not blocked by ergotoxin was (mostly) a relaxation of smooth muscle cells. In the 1940s, Ahlquist in the USA studied different adrenaline-like compounds, and from their different effects correctly postulated the existence of 'alpha' and 'beta' adrenergic receptors. It was realised that drugs acting on the 'beta' receptor might have use in relaxing the constriction of bronchial muscles which is one of the major symptoms of asthma (the other is secretion of mucus). The beta-adrenergic receptor-selective drug isoprenaline had been made by Konzett at the University of Vienna in the late 1930s, and after the Second World War was used to treat asthma. But isoprenaline was found to be very dangerous; there were a number of deaths, probably as a result of stimulant effects on the heart. At this stage, it was realised that there might be two types of beta receptor; one type on the heart, whose activation was undesirable, and one type on the bronchial smooth muscles, whose activation would cause relaxation and thereby assist relieve the bronchoconstriction of asthma. Ultimately, the beta-2 selective drug for relief of asthma became available in the late 1960s, built on the accumulated basic research which had started nearly seventy years earlier.

As I have shown, drug discovery is reliant on basic research. But does that mean that basic research of all types should be allowed to carry on in the hope that ultimately it might generate a new drug? Firstly, it is almost impossible to predict which basic research is going to provide that foundation. Secondly, there is no one correct way to perform experiments on animals. Saying that all use of animals is wrong is an

---

receptor subtype present on voluntary muscles, which is activated by the small neurotransmitter molecule acetylcholine, and then causes an electrical discharge of the muscle cell, which (by downstream mechanisms) then contracts.

over-simplification. There is a wide spectrum of severity of procedures using animals. The impact in terms of pain and distress has to be considered on a case by case basis.

Proponents of the use of animals in biomedical research often say that it is necessary because studies in isolated systems (*in vitro*) cannot mimic the complexity that happens when a drug is given to a living organism. For example, when a drug is taken orally, one must be able to understand how much of it is absorbed from the gastro-intestinal tract, how much of it becomes 'available' in the blood stream (as opposed to either being broken down to inactive molecules, or perhaps being bound to something like a protein), how much of it will reach the target, how long all of this will take, how the drug is eliminated from the body and whether or not the drug or its metabolites have toxic effects (to name but a few). All of this sounds very plausible, but the idea that these sorts of things can only be found from animal studies begs the question of how relevant those studies are to what goes on in humans. As Scarborough and Zalcberg (2017) point out, differences in these regards between animals and humans can thereby be 'benign in one species [and] deadly in another'. The toxic effects of thalidomide (which caused dreadful defects in human embryos – teratogenesis - when their mothers took it for morning sickness) were missed because the animals in which it was initially tested (rats and mice) break the molecule down faster than humans, so resist the toxic effects. Scarborough and Zalcberg give two examples of more modern treatments (TGN1412 for leukaemia; fialuridine for hepatitis B) which killed or nearly killed people in human volunteer (safety) trials, or early clinical tests, because human cells had a particular sensitivity to these molecules which is not present in the test animals.

The main justification for animal experiments is that they are valid because experimental animals are similar to humans. For example, there are numerous claimed animal models of some human diseases. But those who use animals in research often contradict themselves by saying that inflicting cruelty on animals is not so much of a concern because, after all, they are not human.

Critics of animal use in research often express the view that all animal use is wrong. This argument is too simplistic, as it ignores the variability of the impact on the animals involved. Thus, the development of salbutamol, referred to above, initially relied on nothing much more than observation of the responses of a piece of tracheal muscle suspended in a modified saline solution. This tissue would have been taken from a dead guinea-pig. In this case, the justification for killing the animal is no different from the justification for killing an animal to eat it. However, within this argument there remains more than a grain of truth, because animal *models* of human disease more and more frequently have turned out to be anything but.[570] Serious questions have been raised about the ability of a range of animal models to predict efficacy in human disease, including those for antipsychotic activity, antidepressant activity and analgesia. In a very high number of cases, results obtained in animals do not translate to positive results in humans.[571] Perel et al (2007) looked at a range of treatments and diseases in humans, and corresponding work in animal models. They found some reported instances of treatments which were effective in humans (for example, antenatal corticosteroids for respiratory distress in neonates), but not in animals, and some reports of positive effects in animals which did not translate to humans (eg use of corticosteroids for treatment of head injury). The use of transgenic models, where a particular gene is knocked out, or over-expressed, has also seen disappointing results. This may be because the animal with the genetic modification is able to engage compensatory mechanisms.[572] One must

---

[570] see for example Horrobin (2003); Laurijssens et al. (2013) on animal models of Alzheimer's disease; Durham and Blanco (2015); Scarborough and Zalcberg (2017).
[571] Hackam and Redelmeier (2006).
[572] Enna and Williams (2009).

look at so-called animal models of human disease with a very jaundiced and critical eye.

The modern view is that goal-oriented research (as opposed to basic, curiosity-driven research) is best. So grant-awarding bodies will lean towards funding the proposal that aims to find a cure for disease x, y or z. This results in scientists putting up research proposals to try and couch their research (if they can) in terms of a putative benefit, even though the likelihood of such a benefit eventuating may be small. As an example, one frequently sees, in the heartwarming segment following the TV news, scientists claiming that they have made a breakthrough discovery which could lead to a cure for.... (name the disease of choice). In other words, this represents the scientists going outside the system and appealing directly to the non-scientific public, in the hopes of garnering more support for their work.[573] It is relatively easy for a scientist working on a biological system to invent a connection to a supposed medical benefit. The truth is that if one had to prove a justification of basic research by showing a high likelihood of success in terms of medical benefit, most such projects would not succeed in getting approved.

But both goal-oriented research and basic research (if one accepts it can inadvertently provide the foundation for goal-oriented research) face an enormous problem. This is that success in translating any research into medical benefits is becoming less and less likely. If one takes the number of new therapies emerging from the pharmaceutical industry as a benchmark, it is apparent that in recent years there has been a drastic reduction in the rate of significant discoveries resulting in new drugs.[574] The number of new drugs approved per billion US dollars spent on research and development has halved every 9 years since 1950.[575]

---

[573] See the excellent article by Terry Kenakin and others on the situation in biomedical science today: Kenakin et al. (2013); see also Horrobin (2003); Gershell and Atkins (2003).
[574] Durham and Blanco (2015); Bowen and Casadevall (2015).
[575] Scannell et al. (2012).

Even the Food and Drug Administration[576] in the US has noted in a report that 'the current medical product development path is becoming increasingly challenging, inefficient and costly'. It remarks that during the few years leading up to its report (published in 2004) the number of new drug applications declined significantly and notes 'the vast majority of investigational products that enter clinical trials fail'.[577] It is likely that several major drug companies, including Merck Sharp & Dohme, Lilly and Pfizer, will be spending less on research and development, perhaps in response to shareholder pressure.[578] The cost of developing a new drug ranges from US$3.7 billion to US$11.8 billion.[579] This will, one would have thought, reduce the prospects of successful new products even further.[580] This may well be because the technically easy problems have been solved – the so-called 'low-hanging fruit' phenomenon; only the really hard diseases are left.[581] This includes most of the brain disorders, such as Alzheimer's disease and Parkinson's disease[582], and psychiatric disorders such as depression and schizophrenia. It is apparent that various forms of cancer are still a major problem, as are diseases like arthritis. A parallel aspect of this phenomenon is that there are some very effective drugs around which, because they were discovered some time ago, and are no longer covered by patents (ie are available as generic drugs), are quite cheap.[583] Another issue which appears to contribute to the problem is the lack of reproducibility of

---

[576] This entity is responsible for reviewing and approving all new therapeutic drug registration applications.

[577] *Challenges and opportunities report – March 2004* Food & Drug Administration at https://www.fda.gov/ScienceResearch/SpecialTopics/CriticalPathInitiative/.

[578] Scannell et al. (2012).

[579] Kannt and Wieland (2016).

[580] Scannell et al. (2012).

[581] Williams (2011).

[582] In early 2018 Pfizer announced it was stopping research on Alzheimer's disease and Parkinson's disease, after a series of costly failures: *Pfizer abandons research into Alzheimer's and Parkinson's diseases*, BMJ 2018,;360:k122.

[583] Scannell et al. (2012).

research findings.[584] This must be sheeted back to poor review procedures.[585] This is also driven to some extent by the need for researchers to justify themselves in terms of successful publications. It is clear (for example if one looks at the NHMRC as an example) that getting publications is crucial to future grant-winning success. This will serve as a serious impetus for researchers to be less critical than they should be in using proper statistically-valid experimental designs and analysis. Finally, there is the valid complaint that regulatory authorities (of which the FDA is the major one) are said to have become much more stringent in their requirements, so that many drugs fail to pass; moreover, the time taken to develop a drug to the approval stage is now very long: up to 15 years.[586] So it is a long time before companies can get a financial return on their research investment. It is hardly surprising, therefore, that drug companies have decreased in number, with many large-scale mergers. This has in turn resulted in far fewer research jobs, and a move from a research emphasis to an emphasis on marketing and selling the drugs they already have.

Even the success of the human genome project has been questioned. By defining the DNA sequences which code for every gene in humans, this enormous undertaking theoretically opened the door for development of new molecules for disease treatment. However, leading workers are quoted as saying 'the medical benefits derived from the human genome [are] close to zero'.[587] This may be a result of a lack of true understanding of how those molecules work in a native cell (as opposed to an immortalised cell line, which bears no relationship to a normal cell). Furthermore, it appears that many diseases, such as neuropsychiatric conditions (eg schizophrenia) have many discrete

---

[584] see Chapter 4 on problems with statistics in research, and Ritskes-Hotinga and Waver (2018).

[585] Kannt and Wieland (2016).

[586] Kannt and Wieland (2016).

[587] Williams (2011).

causal genetic associations; for example, there seem to be about 70 gene associations with Alzheimer's disease.[588]

Some are even beginning to query the economic viability of research and development in much of the pharmaceutical industry.[589] David Horrobin, writing in 2003, provocatively said *'pharmaceutical research is failing in its ability to deliver new drugs. Furthermore, as much pharmaceutical research draws on the wider biomedical research community, the possibility is that biomedical research in general is also failing'*. For Australian research, that latter statement is the key one.

This overview sets out what I think is the basis on which we should be criticising the use of animals in science. It is not good enough to make some tenuous connection to a disease target when proposing use of animals in research. Given the increasing failure rate in drug discovery, any claimed linkage must be scrutinised carefully. Likewise, given the problem with reproducibility of research findings, project proposals must be subject to criticism of their experimental design by people who know how experiments should be designed. So it is necessary to analyse whether the legal framework allows these criticisms.

### The law governing animal use in teaching and scientific research

The core document governing use of animals in teaching and research is the 8th edition (2013) of the *Australian code for the care and use of animals for scientific purposes*, published by the National Health and Medical Research Council (NHMRC). It has no legal status, but acquires that by being incorporated (in various ways) into States and Territories law.[590]

The Code is based on utilitarian principles, accepting that there must be a balance between the 'potential effects on the wellbeing of animals' used in research, *versus* the 'potential benefits to human, animals or

---

[588] Enna and Williams (2009).
[589] Scannel and Bosley (2015).
[590] See Appendix 8.

the environment'. So the premise is that society accepts that animal use for science is justified, providing there is benefit. The Code covers the use of animals for 'scientific purposes'. It is important to appreciate the breadth of what is permitted under that heading – these are:

> *'all activities conducted with the aim of acquiring, developing or demonstrating knowledge or techniques in all areas of science, including teaching, field trials, environmental studies, research (including the creation and breeding of a new animal line where the impact on animal wellbeing is unknown or uncertain), diagnosis, product testing and the production of biological products'.*

So activities which are expressly allowable include curiosity-driven research, although there must be 'scientific or educational merit' and 'potential benefits' to justify those activities. There is no definition of what 'benefit' means, although projects can only be undertaken 'to obtain and establish significant information relevant to the understanding of humans and/or animals' (amongst other things, including the usual statements about improving human health, etc). The other justifications are improving animal management or production, understanding the natural environment or achieving educational outcomes.

From the animals' point of view, the Code talks about 'the ethical, humane and responsible care and use' of the animals involved. Critically, the Code requires that animal use involves 'scientific integrity'. It expressly requires application of the concepts embodied in the '3Rs', and emphasises the need to avoid or minimise 'harm, including pain and distress'. It covers the use of animals when the aim is to 'acquire, develop or demonstrate knowledge or techniques in any area of science', and extends to activities including 'acquisition, transport, breeding, housing, husbandry, use of animals in a project, and so on'. It is much broader in its reach than the general animal welfare law, extending to the 'care and use of all live non-human vertebrates and cepahalopods'. Likewise, it makes specific reference to the need to take into account an animal's sentience 'and ability to experience pain and distress'. It makes note of the need to be aware of the ontogeny of neural systems enabling this capability, so that institutions must be aware of when procedures using embryos, fetuses and larval forms need to address these questions. It provides a rule of thumb that when such forms are beyond half the gestation or incubation period, or become capable of independent feeding, 'the potential for them to experience pain and distress should be taken into account'.

The Code talks about 'distress', which it defines thus: 'an animal is in a negative mental state and has been unable to adapt to stressors so as to sustain a state of wellbeing'. 'Wellbeing' is said to be where 'an animal is in a positive mental state and is able to achieve successful biological function, to have positive experiences, to express innate behaviours, and to respond to and cope with potentially adverse conditions.' This state can be assessed by 'physiological and behavioural measures of an animal's physical and psychological health and of the animal's capacity to cope with stressors and species-specific behaviours in response to social and environmental conditions'. The Code then says that 'distress' can be 'manifest as abnormal physiological or behavioural responses, a deterioration in physical and psychological health, or a failure to achieve successful biological function. Distress can be acute or chronic and may result in pathological conditions or death'. 'Pain' is also defined, using the definition of pain scientist Alex Iggo: 'an unpleasant sensory and emotional experience associated with actual or potential tissue damage'. There is a whole section (section 3) on 'animal wellbeing'. Animals must be looked after properly; they must be monitored; action must be taken as appropriate; pain and distress must be minimised and so on and so forth. There are specific provisions relating to the relief of pain and distress, using anaesthesia, analgesia and sedation. Animals which have undergone surgery must receive pain relief.

There is a quite remarkable statement in the body of the Code, which again is worth reproducing in full: *'Pain and distress may be difficult to evaluate in animals. Unless there is evidence to the contrary, it must be assumed that procedures and conditions that would cause pain and distress in humans cause pain and distress in animals.'* This is, therefore, a precautionary principle applied to animal welfare, inviting the researcher to actively be anthropomorphic. There is a separate set of guidelines relating to the alleviation of pain and distress.[591]

I set this out more or less *verbatim* so that readers can see that these definitions are far more extensive than any definition in any statute dealing with animal welfare. They clearly encompass the need for animals to have positive sensations, and address issues such as the need to express innate behaviours. These are almost model definitions and in passing I note they clearly highlight the inadequacy of definitions in the animal welfare law dealing with (for example) farm animals.

The Code goes on to express sentiments which reflect the sort of thing said by ethicists.[592] So scientists must have 'respect for animals'. Animal use must be subject to 'ethical review'. They must demonstrate that use of animals is essential to achieve their aims – there must be no suitable non-animal alternatives. There must be minimal impact on animal wellbeing and the minimum number of animals must be used. 'Death as an endpoint' must be avoided unless it is essential to the aims of the project. Methods must be scientifically valid, there must be proper experimental design, and this must include proper statistical analysis. Scientists are under an obligation to research 'existing databases' to consider whether non-animal replacements are available for the proposed research.

---

[591] NHMRC Guidelines to promote the wellbeing of animals used for scientific purposes: the assessment and alleviation of pain and distress in research animals.
[592] See Chapter 3.

Another document worth mentioning is the NHMRC's *Principles and guidelines for the care and use of non-human primates for scientific purposes* (2016). This refers to the 'special ethical and welfare issues' relating to non-human primate use, particularly given they can be used as animal models for human disease 'given their close phylogenetic relationship to humans'. It says 'there is concern that the compromise to their life associated with their confinement and use in scientific research may cause greater psychological suffering than with other species'. No justification is given for this latter statement. I cannot see what this document says which is different from the general statements relating to animal use in the NHMRC Code. The principles are identical: there must be justification, harm must be weighed against potential benefit, and the principles of the 3Rs must be applied at every stage.

The central arbiter of all of this impressive framework is the animal ethics committee. The obligations of institutions where research is carried out include ensuring there is a properly-constituted animal ethics committee (which can, if necessary, be external). The obligations include all the sorts of administrative arrangements you would expect to see (need to monitor, emergency plans, ensuring competence of those involved, etc). Every four years, there must be an 'independent external review'. There is a separate section dealing with this. Amazingly, institutions themselves decide who carries out the review. It is, therefore, self-regulation. The constitution of the animal ethics committee is defined. There must be a chairperson (and the Code hints that it is best if this person comes from the institution), at least one person from each of four categories, being a qualified veterinarian, a person with 'substantial and recent experience in the use of animals for scientific purposes', an animal welfare person (not employed by the institution) and someone from the 'wider community' who has never been involved in scientific animal use, and is not employed by the institution. The latter two classes of person must comprise at least one third of the committee membership. The institution gets to choose the members of the animal ethics committee, and also the number of persons involved. Clearly, it can 'stack' the committee to ensure the outcomes it wants. So, once again, this effectively allows self-regulation.

Thus the Code, despite so much promise, falls at the last and most important hurdle: independent and rigorous enforcement. Unfortunately, by establishing the animal ethics committee as the central arbiter of which procedures are carried out, this potentially marvellous scheme fails completely.

The only possible way to ensure a fair outcome for animals in this sphere is, once again, to have truly independent regulation. There should be independent scientifically qualified reviewers of all aspects of animal use, particularly the review of project proposals. There should be a national body which does this, and it should report detail of projects and how movement towards implementing the 3Rs is achieved. It is, I think, arguable that something like an animal ethics committee can monitor the care and use of animals, with appropriate audit mechanisms. In my view, this does not require the same degree of scientific knowledge and rigour needed to ensure proper review of project proposals. To my mind, the proper review of proposals is essential to ensure that justifications, the 3Rs, and good scientific design and procedure are part of the proposed project. If this is done properly by knowledgeable independent scientists, who really should be employed public servants (ie not aligned with the researchers or their employers), I think there will be a huge beneficial effect in terms of reducing the impact on animals. The scientists involved do not need to be experts in the relevant field (although of course they could consult experts), but must be versed in experimental design and critical appraisal. This is no different from what a good editor of a scientific journal does on a daily basis in considering papers submitted for publication. In this regard one could be encouraged by the guideline published in 2015 by the New South Wales Animal Research Review

Panel on 'high impact research projects'.[593] These projects are said to be those in which animals experience a moderate or large degree of pain and / or distress. The guideline emphasises the need to consider justification either in contributing substantially to advancement of knowledge or the likelihood of translation into practical benefits. There is a recommendation that advice should be taken from someone with specific knowledge of non-animal alternatives. There is a similar statement about access to a specialist statistician regarding issues around experimental design. However, these worthy sentiments will be frustrated by the fact that the guidance is to Animal Ethics Committees, in other words those self-selected, self-regulating bodies which cannot possibly be said to be independent of the institutions they are meant to be overseeing.

The fundamental problem is that the approval of research projects (and that means not just ethical approval, it means approval of funding) is in essence done by peers of the researchers themselves. They are all part of the same clan, and they are not about to commit career suicide by condemning research of their peers. The person whose work you refuse to approve could well be judging your next research grant proposal or application for ethics committee approval. It was always thus. Of course the quandary is that, unless you are close to the research topic concerned, you are not qualified to pass judgment. For example, the Humane Research Australia website has a long list of experiments done in Australian laboratories on primates. There are about 90 published papers listed, going back about 12 years. If it is assumed that the majority of people will approve of scientific experiments on animals, how then, does one make a judgment as to what should be allowed and what should not? As I have already said, you cannot do this just by saying that only experiments which are beneficial to humanity (or to veterinary science) are allowable, because nobody knows whether basic

---

[593] www.animal.ethics.org.au/_data/assets/pdf_file/0010/710893/ARRP-Guideline-24-Consideration-of-high-impact-projects-by-AECs-December-2015.pdf

scientific experiments will or will not be beneficial in that way at some point in the future. One can only hope that scientists sitting in judgment on other scientists will at least be honest and reject proposals which are inadequate in design. And this is unlikely with the current system.

Another point is that animal ethics committees must include several non-scientists in their membership. This creates another set of problems, because it is impossible for people with a non-scientific background to critically evaluate many proposals.

The upshot is that, even with the best will in the world, you are not going to be able to guarantee that science using animals is always good science, or even not repeating earlier work, or just doing the same thing in another species in order to get another scientific paper published. The best you can hope to do is force scientists to justify themselves according to a set of criteria, which is where the '3Rs' come in. Increasing transparency doesn't necessarily help either. Things that sound shocking to a member of the public may in fact be perfectly justifiable from a scientific perspective. Scientists must get better at criticising themselves and honestly communicating what they are doing. It is not good enough to just put up the shutters. All of which is easier said than done, given that scientists are members of an exclusive clique communicating in 'an increasingly arcane langauge'.[594]

The other fact which cannot be ignored is the great scientific tradition, on which most of the scientific literature is founded, involved use of animals. It takes a brave person indeed to break with that tradition. But this is happening where steps are taken to fund science which seeks to move away from animal use. For example, FRAME[595] in the UK, driven by Professor Michael Balls (now its Honorary President), is one such important force for change. The European equivalent which works to

---

[594] quoting Webster (2005).
[595] the Fund for the Replacement of Animals in Medical Experiments; www.frame.org.uk

develop alternatives to animal use, EURL-EVCAM,[596] is also very important in this regard. This must be the way forward. I believe that the more one finds out about the fundamentals of biology and medicine, the more we can use that knowledge to move out of the comfort zone of using animals in experiments and begin to use non-animal systems to ask the same questions. One may even be able to do sensible experiments in humans. But any such change must involve careful analysis of the applicability of non-animal work to the human situation. Cell-based systems are not the entire answer, as there are many well-documented failures.[597] However, what is needed in Australia is real effort towards reducing use of animals in scientific experiments. This must be underpinned by an allocation of research funds for the development and use of non-animal alternatives. The NHMRC should lead in this regard.

The conclusion is that, if one applies consistent criteria to animal use in other areas, today there appears to be ever decreasing justification for animal use in scientific research where that use causes severe harm. This is particularly so where one is talking about basic research justified on the grounds that there may ultimately be some medical benefit at some unspecified future point. While the regulatory system pays lip service to this criticism, it in fact approves continuation of the *status quo*. If Australian governments are serious about replacing animals in scientific experiments, they should make funds available for scientists to develop alternatives.

### Appendix 8    Law relating to scientific animal use

As is typical with the law relating to animal welfare, the law governing use of animals in scientific research is messy and inconsistent. Although the core document is produced by a central agency (the NHMRC), the law is the responsibility of each State and Territory. There is a mix of requirements for personal licences or authorisations, and institutional

---

[596] see https://eurl-evcm.jrc.ec.europa.eu
[597] See Horrobin (2003).

licences. There is a variety of forms of oversight, perhaps the best of which is the arrangement in New South Wales. However, as has been said, the ultimate decision-making power rests with the animal ethics committees, which are appointed by the institutions they are meant to be overseeing. Scientific research involving animal use is therefore self-regulating, in my view.

*ACT:*                                          *Animal Welfare Act 1992*

s22; a personal authorisation is required for breeding or use: s36; institutions (etc) must be licensed: s25; licence is subject to prescribed conditions: s28. *Animal Welfare Regulation 2001* regs 6A, 6B, 7 in essence prescribe compliance with the Code; *Animal Welfare (Australian Code for the Care and Use of Animals for Scientific Purposes) Code of Practice 2014*).

*New South Wales:*                        *Animal Research Act 1985*

Corporations must be accredited in order to carry out animal research: Part 4, Division 1; section 46. Individuals must be authorised and must carry out research in accordance with the directions of an animal ethics committee: Part 4, Division 3; s47: There is oversight by an Animal Research Review Panel (Part 2). The Act contemplates creation of Animal Ethics Committees, which makes recommendations regarding grant of authorities, and works according to the NHMRC Code (Part 3). Animal suppliers must be licensed: Part 4, Division 5. There are powers of inspection: Part 6.

*Northern Territory:*                      *Animal Welfare Act 1999*

Part 5. Premises must be licensed. It is a condition of the licence that there should be an animal ethics committee: s34(1)(a). A person employed or engaged by a licensee may conduct teaching or research using animals only with a permit: s43(1). Permit holder must comply with Code: s 48(2)(d).

*Queensland:*                          *Animal Care and Protection Act 2001*

Chapter 4. A person must be registered to use an animal for a scientific purpose (or must be retained by a registered person, or be a student at a registered institution). The Code must be complied with: s55(1); s 91 (re animal ethics committee approval).

*South Australia:*                        *Animal Welfare Act 1985*

Part 4. A person must have a licence; an employee of a licensee is not required to have a licence. A licensee must set up an animal ethics committee and research must be done in compliance with the Code: s19 (also Division 2 re animal ethics committees).

*Tasmania:*                             *Animal Welfare Act 1993*

Part 4. Institutions must be licensed. There must be an animal ethics committee and research must be done in accordance with the Code: s30.

*Victoria:*                            *Prevention of Cruelty to Animals Act 1986*

Part 3. A person occupying relevant scientific premises must be licensed: s26; s29; s30. Field work must be licensed, or authorised by a licence holder: s27. Compliance with the Code, and animal ethics committees are dealt with by *Prevention of Cruelty to Animals Regulations 2008*, Part 4.

*Western Australia:*                 *Animal Welfare Act 2002*

Part 2. Institutions are licensed; employees or students at a licensed establishment do not require a licence. There must be an animal ethics committee and animals must be used in accordance with the Code: s6 (also s9).

# Chapter 9    Animals in entertainment

The history of animals and entertainment is horrific. It does seem as if humanity has a fascination with watching animals fighting, performing tricks, being used for 'sport', or being paraded around. Sources on the subject provide detail of the use of wild animals as part of public spectacle in Greek and Roman times. This included ceremonial processions and of course the notorious gladiatorial competitions. Showing off exotic animals such as elephants and lions, was seen as indicative of the high status of whichever notable was involved. In mediaeval times, performing and wild animals were regularly seen at fairs, and the itinerant animal show of the circus became popular, as did the travelling dancing bear, dog or horse.[598] The early animal activists battled in the English parliament with the hugely popular public entertainments of dog fighting, cock fighting and bull-baiting. One could fool oneself that these sorts of revolting pursuits are historical. Not so. In recent years, there has been increasing focus on problems relating to animals in entertainment. Dark practices involving live baiting of greyhounds have long been suspected, but were only exposed in their full horror as recently as 2015. And while this is what is seen above the surface, it is very likely that fights between animals, particularly dogs and roosters, is more common than we would like to think.[599]

That said, it is not all bad news. There have been significant developments concerning the use of whips in horse racing. There has also been some progress in the regulation of rodeos.

In Australia it is not acceptable to celebrate pursuits in which animals are deliberately caused harm for entertainment. It is therefore not surprising that proponents of keeping animals in zoos seek various justifications for what they do. So, for example, zoos claim that they

---

[598] Wilson (2015).
[599] See for example http://www.adelaidenow.com.au/news/south-australia/dogfighting-ring-smashed-after-man-becomes-first-south-australian-charged-over-shocking-blood-sport/news-story/69a31a297745fd2a458d2ad0454fd2f6.

serve an educational purpose, and that they assist in preventing extinctions of species which are threatened.[600] Neither of these claims can possibly justify the actuality of what a zoo is, which is a collection of animals forcibly taken from their natural environment and confined in an artificial environment. Furthermore, animals held captive in zoos are forced to endure incursions by spectators, which are necessarily stressful.[601]

I think there is a reasonable argument that circuses and rodeo represent the last vestiges of the Romans' brutal use of animals for entertainment. So far as circuses are concerned, Clive Phillips has commented that circuses have been reported as using cruel methods to train animals, and notes that animals in circuses are forced to perform in ways that belittles them. He believes (and I agree) that this damages the relationship between humanity and animals. Critics of the concept of animals having 'dignity' perhaps miss the point that, while it is unlikely that animals themselves have a concept of their own dignity, it is not unreasonable for humans to treat animals as if they do have dignity. All this means is having respect for their very nature as animals, rather than forcing them into situations which are contrary to their nature.[602] This is neatly summarised by a report in 2016 for the Welsh Government, which said '...the education and conservation role of travelling circuses and mobile zoos is likely to be marginal, and any potential educational and conservation benefits are likely to be outweighed by the negative impression generated by using wild animals for entertainment'.[603] RSPCA Australia is opposed to the use of wild exotic animals in circuses, as the requirements of animals kept for circuses is not compatible with the animals' physiological, social and behavioural needs. This is because they are kept for lengthy periods in close confinement, held in artificial social groups, and spend much time being transported from site to site.

---

[600] Phillips (2017).
[601] See for example Bonnie et al. (2016), concerning chimpanzees and gorillas in zoos.
[602] Kiley-Worthington (2016).
[603] Dorning et al.(2016).

RSPCA Australia reports that many local councils have prohibited circuses which use exotic animals.[604] Phillips (2017) points out that the popularity of circuses is decreasing, probably because of strong criticism from animal advocacy groups.

The topic is well covered by Alex Bruce.[605]

## Horses

It is apparent that untrained horses do not allow themselves to be ridden. Horses have to be 'broken' to accept a rider. That word means what it says. Breaking a horse can often involve very harsh treatment; but it need not.[606] Training is involved in many aspects of horse use, for example in getting them to go into starting gates for racing, or training them to go over jumps, or carry out the exercises in dressage. In all cases, there is the opportunity for cruel practices, although equally there are many techniques which do not involve cruelty. As eloquently stated by McLean and McGreevy (2010) horse riding involves exploitation different from confining an animal in a cage or pen, but nevertheless involves gaining complete control over the animal's mobility. This gives rise, they say, to a moral responsibility to treat the domestic horse with regard for its welfare. However, they note that there is a particular worry, as it is possible that what appears to be acceptance by a horse of training may in fact amount to learned helplessness. This is a matter for great concern, particularly when one acknowledges that the basis of horse training is negative reinforcement (that is, the avoidance of unpleasant experiences). It is equally valid to say that ethical training and riding is effectively environmental and behavioural enrichment.

---

[604] see kb.rspca.org.au/what-is-the-rspcas-view-on-the-use-of-animals-in-circuses_146.html; see also Part 5 of the *Animal Welfare Act 1992* (ACT) which prohibits the use of bears, elephants, giraffes, primates or felines (other than domestic cats) in a circus.
[605] Bruce (2012).
[606] Broom and Fraser (2007).

### Horse racing

Unlike the situation with circuses, zoos and other use of animals in entertainment, racing of dogs and horses is driven primarily by the gambling industry which is inextricably interwoven with these activities. Huge amounts of money are at stake and as such those involved are surely tempted to be less than ethical in the way the animals used are dealt with. Betting is primarily what has driven regulation in the past, as the potential to make or lose vast sums of money stimulates innovative ways of cheating. Animal welfare has not, in the main, been a driving factor, but has been more of an indirect beneficiary through regulation of activities such as doping and other versions of gaining an unfair advantage.

Horse racing is the dominant form of the 'sport'. In Australia, there are nearly 20,000 races each year, on about 400 tracks, involving just over 35,000 horses. The prize money alone amounts to over half a billion dollars each year. Nearly 18 billion dollars is bet on horse races (that is, flat and harness races) each year.[607]

Horse racing consists of flat and jumps racing (the horses concerned are the breed called 'Thoroughbreds') and trotting or pacing (where the breed is the Standardbred). The latter involves specially trained horses which tow a small cart on which the driver sits. In recent years there has been much criticism of these events, focusing primarily on the use of whips and the high risk of injury or death to horses involved in jumps racing.[608] Groups such as the Coalition for the Protection of Racehorses have brought many of these issues to the attention of the public.[609] At the moment, jumps racing is allowed only in Victoria and South Australia. As pointed out by RSPCA South Australia, in 1991 the Senate Select Committee on Animal Welfare, reporting on the racing industry, expressed serious concerns about the welfare of horses in jumps races, and took the view that it should be phased out over three years. A

---

[607] Racing Australia *Racing Season 2015/2016 Fact Book*.
[608] see McLean and McGreevy (2010).
[609] www.horseracingkills.com.

survey carried out by RPSCA South Australia in 2009 found that only 14% of respondents supported jumps racing.[610]

Racing Australia is the peak body governing horse racing in this country. It establishes the Rules of Racing and its members are the states and territories racing authorities. It has rules which in some regards seek to maintain horse welfare,[611] including rules regarding the use of whips.

Australia is at the forefront of equine behaviour research, through the work of Professor Paul McGreevy of the University of Sydney, and Dr Andrew McLean of the Australian Equine Behaviour Centre. Together with others, these authors have been very influential in establishing equitation science as the basis for changes in horse riding and training.

A perennial problem for the racing industry is the fate of horses which are unsuccessful. The perception is that many horses fail, and are killed as a result. A survey of the horse racing industry found that about 40% of horses left racing stables in the 2002-2003 racing year for reasons including illness, poor performance and unsuitable temperament.[612] The authors estimated that this meant about 15,000 horses might have left the industry in that time (although this was probably an underestimate, as it did not consider horses yet to start in a race). Significant numbers of horses which no longer raced were auctioned, and it is likely that many of these were sent to slaughter. It appeared that about 1500 horses were slaughtered in the study period.

There have been industry initiatives designed to assuage the public concern over failed racehorses being sent to knackeries. In New South Wales, for example, the governing body, Racing NSW, has said every

---

[610] see www.theillogicalraces.org.au/the-issues/why-jumps-racing-is-illogical/
[611] see www.racingaustralia.horse/arb/welfare-guidelines-for-australian-thoroughbred-horseracing.aspx
[612] Thomson et al.(2014).

such horse will be rehomed, in a scheme to take 1% of race prize money to invest in rehabilitation programmes.[613]

Whipping of racehorses is also of concern to the racing industry. The work of Paul McGreevy has undoubtedly played an important part in raising questions about whether using whips on horses is justified. Whipping horses is said to produce the 'best performance' during a race. However, the scientific evidence does not show this.[614] Moreover, there is good evidence that hitting a horse even with a padded whip is probably painful. RSPCA Australia is opposed to the use of whips on racehorses.

Hood et al. (2017) looked at data from racing authorities in New South Wales and the ACT in order to characterise whip use. The records of racing authorities showed breaches of the rules regarding whip use in about 1% of starts. This contrasts with earlier work showing breaches in 6% of starts. The authors suggested that there be closer monitoring of compliance with whip use rules.

Even the horse racing industry is acknowledging there is a problem and that a ban on whips may be inevitable.[615] In harness racing, the industry body, Australian Harness Racing, announced that whips would be banned from 1 September 2017. However, in response to a significant backlash from the industry, that body has watered this down to an undertaking that whips must be used with only a wrist action.[616]

### Horse riding

It could be said that concern for horse welfare was a major driver for the first animal cruelty legislation in England in the 1820s. Moreover, it

---

[613] Andrew Clennell, 'Racing NSW vows to rehome every racehorse in wake of greyhounds shutdown'. *Daily Telegraph* 6 September 2016.

[614] See for example McGreevy et al.(2012).

[615] 'Whip ban inevitable'; racenet 5 January 2017, www.m.racenet.com.au/news/129994/OPINION:-SteveMoran – Whip ban inevitable.

[616] see https://www.harness.org.au/media-room/whip-free-racing/.

could also be said that Anna Sewell's book *Black Beauty* (published in 1877) had as much impact regarding its subject as did Ruth Harrison's book on factory farming nearly a century later.

There is very little information on the number of horses which are kept in Australia and which are not involved in horse racing or other commercial uses. There is no central registry and in any case there is no requirement to register horses. This is quite surprising, as horses are valuable animals, and expensive to keep and maintain. One would have thought a registration system would be very useful, particularly when it comes to buying and selling horses. Furthermore, when there are outbreaks of serious disease, such as recently occurred with equine influenza, one would have thought it would be very useful to know where horses are and who owns them.

Equestrian Australia says it has about 20,000 members, while Pony Club Australia says there are about 27,000 members of pony clubs around the country. However, I think that is an under-estimate of the number of horses. Many people have more than one horse, and many horse riders are not members of associations. An article linked from the Racing Australia website refers to research in 2001 indicating that there are 57,000 horses used for recreation.[617] Although this is old data, it may provide a better estimate of current numbers.

Horse riding is very much big business. One only has to look at a horse magazine to see how much money can cheerfully be spent on keeping horses. The two associations I mentioned in the previous paragraph do a good job of educating their members in horse welfare, which is a very complex area. Because feeding horses can result in substantial costs, it is often the case that uncaring owners allow horses to starve, either by not providing enough access to feed in a paddock, or otherwise supplementing feed. Horses can get sick very easily and veterinary treatment is expensive and often difficult. They can be hard to transport

---

[617] pateblog.nma.gov.au/2014/10/01/what-happens-to-all-those-racehorses/

– and of course horse floats are themselves very expensive. They need to have their hooves trimmed regularly by expert practitioners (farriers) and require specialist dental treatment.[618]

Riding horses for pleasure, or for events such as dressage, showjumping, or riding cross country, can be associated with significant welfare problems. For example, in dressage, there has been a tendency to using extreme bending of the neck ('cervical hyperflexion') as a training aid. But this itself represents an underlying issue which should be avoided which is the application of too much pressure on the horse's bit. Indeed, there is a good argument for altering dressage rules to give more marks for horses which perform with the (apparent) minimum of interference from the rider.[619]

I confess I am equivocal about horse riding. It is very easy to get fond of horses, but I do wonder whether it is the best thing (for them) to ride them. Having said that, this is another one of those things that is not going to change in a hurry, so the best one can do is to advocate for the best possible outcomes for the animals.

### Greyhound racing[620]

Australia is one of a very small number of countries which allows greyhound racing.[621] Like horse racing, greyhound racing is driven by betting.[622] For example, in 2015, over 1 billion dollars was wagered on greyhound racing in New South Wales alone; greyhound racing in New South Wales and Victoria constitute the largest involvement of the so-called sport in Australia. It is quite likely that this focus on betting shifts

---

[618] see Broom and Fraser (2007).

[619] McLean and McGreevy (2010).

[620] The following is based on McHugh (2016).

[621] Other jurisdictions which allow greyhound racing are Mexico, Macau, New Zealand, Eire, the UK and Vietnam.

[622] Greyhound racing may comprise about 20% of betting turnover in New South Wales. The total amount wagered and bet on greyhound racing in 2015-16 was just over 3 billion dollars: Racing Australia *Racing Season 2015/2016 Fact Book.*

the focus away from animal welfare concerns, as wagerers are quite dissociated from the activity; only a minority attend race meetings. Regarding non-betting financial benefit of greyhound racing, in financial year 2013 it was said (by one report) to have generated nearly $350 million in direct and indirect financial benefit to New South Wales alone. However, another report which was produced a few years earlier indicated that these figures may be exaggerated by about 3-fold, and the McHugh inquiry regarded both of these figures as too high.

Until 2015 the greyhound racing industry was not regarded as especially troublesome. There was a report commissioned by the Victorian government in 2008 and a 2014 Select Committee inquiry conducted by the parliament of New South Wales, both of which raised concerns about the number of dogs which seemingly disappeared from the industry ('wastage' – see below), but all in all the concerns were at the level of suspicions rather than anything tangible. This changed in 2015, when undercover footage, taken initially by Animal Liberation Queensland, revealed what appeared to be the extensive use of live animals as lures to train greyhounds. As with the 2011 live export revelations, Animals Australia and the ABC's *Four Corners* was front and centre in this exposure.[623] The saddest aspect of this is that, once again, not only was a major part of an industry regularly using a criminal practice involving high levels of cruelty to animals, but the agency responsible for protecting animal welfare had turned a blind eye to it. To those interested in animal welfare matters, this is a depressingly familiar scenario. It took the brave (and illegal) actions of some ordinary citizens, coupled with bold journalism, to prompt action. In fact the regulator was well aware of the implications of these practices coming to the attention of the public. Some of its documents, created well before the revelations, made prescient reference to any such exposure allowing 'growing welfare extremists' (*sic*) to force change in racing codes. The use of that phrase of course illustrates how such regulatory bodies, charged with looking after the welfare of animals, regard

---

[623] 16 February 2015 *Making a killing.*

anybody else with concern for the animals as 'extremists'. This, I think, neatly summarises the wider problem in Australia today.

Government inquiries were initiated in several states,[624] but the New South Wales inquiry, under Michael McHugh (formerly of the High Court), was far and away the most comprehensive and useful. So far as animal welfare is concerned, it was ground-breaking, in that it expressly acknowledged that operations of this sort were not conducted merely for the benefits of participants (wagerers, employees, audiences, and so on), but that the public in general had a stake. It discussed at length the nature of this 'social licence'. It noted it was not a legal term, but rather was something related to whether there was 'integrity-based trust'. It was also unwaveringly critical of Greyhound Racing New South Wales (GRNSW), the government body charged with overseeing the industry. It was clear that body was in essence corrupt, in that its senior managers were aware of many of the practices under investigation, but did nothing.

The use of live baiting, involving fastening rabbits, possums and piglets to lures and allowing dogs to chase, maul and kill the live animals, was what prompted the inquiry. The practice was clearly prevalent in the industry (and had been for some time), and was believed by its perpetrators to give their dogs a competitive advantage. In this respect, it was not only heinous animal abuse, it was a fraud on those who obeyed the rules. As noted by the inquiry, the practice, along with hare coursing, had specifically been made illegal in 1967, and continued to be illegal under section 21 of the New South Wales *Prevention of Cruelty to Animals Act 1997*. The worst aspect of the evidence found by the

---

[624] Tasmania: Joint Select Committee on Greyhound Racing in Tasmania *Final Report: Review of Arrangements for Animal Welfare in the Tasmanian Greyhound Racing Industry*, 13 March 2015; Victoria: *2015 Own Motion Inquiry into Live Baiting in Greyhound Racing in Victoria Final Report* (Office of the Racing Integrity Commissioner); *Investigation into Animal Welfare and Cruelty in the Victorian Greyhound Industry*, 30 April 2015 (Dr Charles Milne, Chief Veterinary Officer); Queensland: the MacSporran Report, 1 June 2015.

inquiry was that several trainers in the industry aggressively refused to accept there was anything wrong with the practice. This also illustrates what has long been suspected about greyhound racing – that it attracts an element which could best be described as violent and criminal.

The McHugh inquiry looked at all aspects of the greyhound racing 'industry', examining not only the practice of live baiting, but other issues, including 'wastage' of animals. In this regard, the inquiry calculated that in a 12 year period, between about 40,000 and 70,000 animals were deliberately killed because they weren't good enough. It was difficult to be more precise, because GRNSW did not keep appropriate records. There was very little rehoming. The inquiry concluded that this 'wastage' was unsustainable. This in itself is interesting, because, like all animals which are owned, there is nothing to stop a greyhound owner killing the animal. It is not illegal. So why the concern? According to the inquiry, 'wastage...has attracted attention for decades. It has led some to question whether greyhound racing should have any place in a modern civilised society. This is unsurprising'. The inquiry came close to explaining that concern when, after noting that it was not illegal to kill dogs which were no good, it remarked in effect that doing business in this way would not be consistent with the industry's 'social licence'. In other words, there is a complete disjunction between what the law permits and what the public is prepared to accept. The 'wastage' was said to be 'at odds with the animal welfare expectations of modern Australians and would be repugnant to many of them'.

Another fascinating issue turned up by the inquiry was the sanitising of public reports of racing by GRNSW in order to hide the number of greyhounds killed or injured during races. The concern was that telling the truth would 'stir up the greenies'. The regulatory authority thereby seemed to be operating a policy of seeking to hide the truth from the public. The data obtained by the inquiry indicated that over 20% of greyhounds competing in a year would suffer an injury, over 4% of which could be described as 'major or catastrophic'. Moreover, it was apparent that many owners and trainers of greyhounds would virtually never consult a veterinarian when a dog was injured. They maintained an arrogant self-confidence that they knew what was best and were extremely reluctant to spend money on the dogs in any case. Much of the treatment involved bizarre interventions by unqualified individuals, with the sole intention of enabling the dog to race, rather than ensuring injuries were properly treated. Much of these so-called treatments are themselves extremely painful.[625] Finally, the inquiry condemned the practice of exporting greyhounds to race in places such as Macau where animal welfare standards are absent.

The inquiry recommended that the New South Wales parliament should consider whether greyhound racing should be allowed to continue. It expressed the view that while effective policing of the industry could greatly reduce if not eliminate the practice of live baiting, it would be unlikely that the industry would be able to do anything about the level of 'wastage' of dogs in the industry. It made 80 recommendations for change in the event a decision was made to allow the industry to continue. In July 2015, Mike Baird, the New South Wales Premier, announced an end to greyhound racing in the State. In August 2015, the New South Wales Parliament passed a law to this effect. The backlash commenced immediately, and it was ferocious. The Labor Party opposed the ban and several Nationals MPs voted against the legislation. The then federal Nationals leader, Barnaby Joyce, was very outspoken against the ban. In an ironic twist, arguments against banning greyhound racing included that it was depriving poorer people of their entertainment (the irony is that this is exactly the same argument mounted against those proposing animal welfare legislation in the English parliament in the 1820s, where the concern was that bull-baiting and the like would be banned). Subsequently, Liberals did badly in New South Wales local council elections and polls showed that the

---

[625] Examples included self-treatment of broken limbs, injection of vitamins, and the employment of so-called 'muscle men', who are unqualified persons who claim to be knowledgeable about treatment of ailments in greyhounds.

ban was badly received by the public.[626] By October 2016, Baird was saying he had made a mistake, and the ban was going to be reversed. This appeared to be based on a report on the industry by Dr John Keniry, which indicated that reforms could achieve real change. By the beginning of 2017, Baird had resigned as Premier.[627]

In reversing the ban, the New South Wales government in October 2016 set up the Greyhound Industry Reform Panel to provide recommendations on animal welfare and the way the industry is run. This group made recommendations it said were 'broadly consistent' with those of the McHugh inquiry.[628] The main recommendation was that the commercial and regulatory functions of the regulator at the time of the reported incidents, GRNSW, be separated. In response to this, in May 2017 the government announced it would be establishing an independent Greyhound Welfare and Integrity Commission. This is contemplated by the *Greyhound Racing Act 2017*, which is yet to commence in full. However, the government has placed advertisements for the Commissioners.[629] The new Act includes the establishment of a Greyhound Industry Animal Welfare Committee, whose membership will include a person with animal welfare or animal behaviour expertise. There will also be a code of practice, with certain provisions which must be complied with. There will be a life ban for those involved in the industry who commit a 'live baiting offence'. These are all changes for the better.

---

[626] see www.abc.net.au/news/2016-10-11/everything-you-need-to-know-about-mike-baird-greyhounds/7921306

[627] Gerathy, Sarah (2016). *Mike Baird: how NSW Premier went from popular to political scrapheap.* www.abc.net.au/news/2017-01-19/mike-baird-resigns-how-mr-popular-ended-up-on-the-scrapheap/81936

[628] Recommendations of the Greyhound Industry Reform Panel (2017); see www.industry.new.gov.au/about/our-business/department/racing/greyhound-racing

[629] Former NSW premier Morris Iemma was appointed as the first Commissioner.

The conclusion of all of this is, despite the unfortunate demise of New South Wales Premier Baird, the legislative and governance changes put in place may have the effect of greatly improving animal welfare in greyhound racing. This remains to be seen.

## Rodeos

Rodeos originated in the USA, but apparently made an appearance in Australia in 1888. Rodeo enjoys some popularity in Australia, particularly in country areas. Amongst other things, it involves riding horses or bulls which basically do not want to be ridden. The 'fun' is in seeing how long the rider can stay on the frantic and panicked animal. Other 'skills' on display in rodeos include calf roping. This is done by someone on horseback pursuing a petrified calf, which is roped around the neck, after which the rider dismounts and throws the calf to the ground. Another attraction is where a horse rider chases a bull, leaps from the horse, grabs the bull by the horns and wrestles it to the ground. So this is entertainment in which animals are harassed and terrorised, with a test of the strength of the participants. It's a bit like biting the heads off live rats, only on a larger scale, but equally stupid.

It seems evident that many of these events, involving animals which are very scared, involve a compromise of the animals' welfare. Clive Phillips' group has shown that roped calves show a marked increase in cortisol, adrenaline and noradrenaline after roping, consistent with their being heavily stressed. However, the authors note some problems with their study, including the perennial problem of when it is best to sample to best detect changes in cortisol.[630]

RSPCA Australia opposes rodeos because of what it says is the potential for significant injury, suffering and distress. It highlights the particular problem of calf roping, saying that animals can suddenly be jerked by the rope around the neck, and can be dragged along the ground. Likewise the throwing of the animal to the ground is a cause for

---

[630] Sinclair et al.(2016).

concern. The Australian Veterinary Association is not opposed to rodeos, but nevertheless notes that 'there is considerable inherent welfare risk to animals participating in rodeos'. It remarks that many rodeos, particularly in out of the way places, are not properly regulated. Rodeos are tightly regulated in Victoria, under the *Prevention of Cruelty to Animals Regulations 2008*, Part 3. Rodeos must be licenced and have a veterinarian in attendance. Calf roping is not permitted in practical terms, as animals which weigh less than 200 kilograms cannot be used. Rodeos are prohibited in the ACT. The South Australian *Animal Welfare Act* 1985 requires rodeos to be licenced, and like Victoria, the subordinate legislation allows only adult animals to be used, amounting to a *de facto* ban on calf roping. In Tasmania, rodeos must be conducted in accordance with the NCCAW Standards (s11A *Animal Welfare Act* 1993), which include a requirement for a veterinarian to be in attendance. In New South Wales, animals involved in rodeos are exempted from the provisions of the *Exhibited Animals Protection Act 1986* by regulation 5 of the cognate regulations. Rodeos are also exempted from the prohibitions in sections 18, 18A and 20 of the *Prevention of Cruelty to Animals Act 1979* (relating to animal baiting, bull fighting, causing an animal to fight) by regulation 36 of the *Prevention of Cruelty to Animals Regulation 2012*.

What all of this means is that in Australia, as with hunting, in rodeo we have another vestigial testosterone-fuelled display of masculine aggression, passing as entertainment, and vigorously defended by its participants as 'part of their culture'. I have little hope there will be change for the better in the foreseeable future. As ever, all one can hope to do is minimise the damage to the animals forced to participate in this 'entertainment'.

# Chapter 10  Killing animals for fun, and commercial hunting

## Killing animals for fun[631]

Hunting for pleasure (as opposed to survival – rare these days) is the ultimate denial of the intrinsic value of an animal.

The choice of the title for this section is deliberate. I am sure many people regard 'hunting' as something that is done for reasons other than for the fun of killing an animal, or perhaps don't even think about it. Defenders of hunting often camouflage the practice with justifications which distract from the reality. They will talk about gathering food, preserving environment, adding commercial value, ridding us of unwanted pests, keeping rampant animal population growth under control, and the justification of such practices because they have cultural significance.[632] Some of the wackier justifications include that hunters achieve a sort of transcendental or spiritual higher state; some are even prepared to admit to hunting providing an outlet for men's sexual energy.[633] These are all euphemisms for killing for fun. That is, I think, the definition of sadism. Hunters will even try and maintain that, were it not for them, animals would suffer terribly, because after all, life is terribly tough in the wild.[634] But one thing hunters rarely admit to is that they enjoy killing things, presumably because they know the majority of people would find that unacceptable. There are exceptions; Kheel (1996) quotes Ernest Hemingway as saying 'I think birds were made to be shot and some of us were made to shoot them and if that is not so well, never say we did not tell you that we like it'. At least he was being honest. As ever, John Webster cuts through the nonsense, saying '*I am on the side of those*

---

[631] for a measured review of this topic, see Thiriet (2009).
[632] see Kheel (1996); Thiriet (2009).
[633] Kheel (1996).
[634] see Plous (2002).

*who feel the whole concept of killing animals for pleasure to be morally objectionable'.*[635]

Hunting is as old as the human species, one suspects. As civilisation progressed, hunting for fun, as opposed to for food, became highly regarded as a pastime for noble classes.[636] Killing an animal for 'sport' should be roundly condemned by thinking persons. Indeed, the description of hunting as a 'sport' is misleading, as the other participant in the 'sport' (that is, the unfortunate animal being hunted) hardly has a choice in the matter.[637]

The other factor which must be steadily borne in mind is that hunting, from early days a male preserve, itself evolved into something which promoted the traits of masculinity said to be desirable. Kheel (1996) notes that there were early arguments that hunting 'was a necessary corrective for men who had become overtly feminized by the encroaches of civilization'. Sport hunting was a 'necessary release for man's instinctual and aggressive drives'. That more or less says it all.

What is clear is that hunting animals for whatever reason is incompatible with good animal welfare. Not only is killing a sentient animal for fun the taking and wasting of a life for pleasure, it is virtually impossible to do in a humane manner. Where amateurs are involved, there is a strong likelihood that animals being hunted will be terrorised, wounded and traumatised, rather than being killed cleanly or humanely. Moreover, the negative effect of killing individuals on the social structure of animals which live in groups can be significant.[638]

One doesn't need to be a psychologist or sociologist to know that there is still a substantial number of people who get a kick out of seeing animals suffer, or killing them. It would not seem unreasonable to

---

[635] Webster (2005).
[636] Griffin (2007).
[637] Kheel (1996).
[638] Thiriet (2009).

suggest this is a very basic human trait. Indeed, it should be recalled that the very first attempts to create laws to reduce animal cruelty in England were aimed at 'sports' like bull-baiting (see Chapter 5). It was ironic that during the recent heated debate about cruelty in the greyhound racing industry (using live animals as baits) one of the complaints against those seeking to ban the 'sport' was that it would unreasonably penalise 'ordinary people'. These were exactly the same arguments which were being raised against Richard Martin MP in the English Parliament in the 1820s. The corollary of that argument, of course, is that 'ordinary people', if the argument is correct, are more sadistic than people who are not 'ordinary'. This has about as much moral weight as governments justifying their failure to ban smoking because it is a pleasure of the ordinary person which they must be allowed. If the 'ordinary person' thinks that killing animals for pleasure is a good thing, then they need to be educated otherwise. Personally, I think the 'ordinary person' argument is a political smokescreen.

The conflict between what is acceptable and what is unacceptable in pursuing, torturing and killing animals for pleasure is evident in the legislation. Animal baiting, cockfighting and dog fights, all of which were popular 'sports', are all banned; even possession of relevant paraphernalia is also an offence in some jurisdictions.[639] But hunting is permitted, providing a person has the relevant authorisations, licences and so on, although of course owners of farming land can kill animals without any such authorisation, in the main. The moral figleaf extends to seeking to regulate the use of dogs in hunting, whereby dogs cannot be used to attack animals, such as pigs. For example in New South Wales, mandatory provisions of a 'code of practice' (which code does not seem to be published anywhere) include an 'obligation to avoid suffering' and an obligation to locate and kill a wounded animal.[640]

---

[639] for example, ss18, 18A, 21 *Prevention of Cruelty to Animals Act 1979* (NSW); ss14(5), 14A(1)(a) *Animal Welfare Act 1985* (SA); s14 *Prevention of Cruelty to Animals Act 1986* (Vic); Part 3 *Animal Care and Protection Act 2001 Qld)*;
[640] See for example Part 9 of the *National Parks and Wildlife Act 1974* (NSW), which allows the grant of licences allowing a person to 'harm' protected fauna

These provisions are in my view pure fantasy. Preventing people from using dogs to attack hunted animals would be impossible to police, and the idea that hunters are going to concern themselves with tracking down and killing wounded animals, or 'targeting animals so that a humane kill is likely' is window dressing at best. Furthermore, as Thiriet (2009) points out, persons not required to have a licence, which includes those hunting feral animals on private land, do not have to comply with these provisions in any case.

I do not propose to go through the detail of the law concerning the licensing of killing animals for fun, if only because it is a futile and irrelevant exercise. As the example of New South Wales illustrates, even where a licence is required, the provisions regarding animal welfare are unenforceable, unenforced and easily circumvented. The bottom line is if you want to go out and kill animals, you will be able to do it easily and in the main you will be virtually unsupervised. As an example, the practice of using dogs to hunt pigs is widely and openly pursued Australia-wide.

'Recreational' hunting of duck and quail has been banned in Western Australia, New South Wales and Queensland. The first two jurisdictions have also banned goose hunting.[641] In Victoria, given recent success of animal activists (Laurie Levy and Lynn Trakell have been at the forefront) in bringing to light the immorality of duck hunting, the government has reacted by making it an offence for someone to go into a 'specified hunting area' or to approach a person who is hunting or to

---

(s5 defines 'harm' to include hunt); licences for hunting game and feral animals are granted under Part 3 of the *Game and Feral Animal Control Act 2002* (NSW), although there are extensive exemptions for people killing animals on their own land, or on an employer's land (s17) and of course the usual list of non-indigenous animals (Part 2, Schedule 3); as to regulation of hunting, see *Game and Feral Animal Control Regulation 2012* (NSW) Part 3, and Schedule 1 (conditions of licences) and Schedule 2 (mandatory provisions of code of practice).
[641] s15A *Wildlife Conservation Act 1950* (WA); s120(2A) and 120(2C) *National Parks and Wildlife Act 1974* (NSW); s97A *Nature Conservation Act 1992* (Qld).

'hinder or obstruct hunting'.[642] This represents a serious retrograde step. But so far as killing animals for fun is concerned, one has to ask 'what is the difference between baiting and so on, and hunting?'.

The key point is that a significant number of people regard hunting as immoral. When enough people in a society regard something as immoral, then the rest of society, who happen to disagree with that, must conform with the will of the majority. At the moment, Australia has still to achieve an average level of moral awareness such that politicians could feel sufficiently emboldened to take on the hunting issue. So what we are left with is the usual unsatisfactory pretence of purporting to make the activity 'humane'. However, the very act of allowing hunting means that its victims are treated inhumanely. I have often reflected on the impossibility of policing hunting – who in their right mind would want to be out in the middle of the night trying to monitor a group of people armed with guns out to shoot animals? Those who are charged with policing this charade are usually nowhere to be seen. This is illustrated by the following: at the hearing before the Administrative Appeals Tribunal in which Animal Liberation sought to knock down the New South Wales Kangaroo Management Plan, Peter Singleton (barrister for the applicant) managed to get the person in the Department who was responsible for overseeing shooting of kangaroos to admit that everybody in the Department went home at 5pm; that same person then quite cheerfully agreed that the shooting was done in the early hours of the morning.[643]

It is difficult to get figures on how many people are involved in hunting for fun, other than fishing, in Australia. Eleonora Gullone (2015) referenced the figures from www.gunpolicy.org; they currently show that 3.55% of the Australian population are licensed gun owners. Of course, not all of these will engage in hunting as such. Franklin's survey

---

[642] ss58C, 58D and58E *Wildlife Act 1975* (Vic).
[643] *Re Wildlife Protection Association of Australia Inc. and Minister for the Environment, Heritage and the Arts* [2008] AATA 717.

(2007b) indicated that 95% of people had never hunted feral animals, and 99% of people had never hunted native wildlife. As Gullone (2015) says, all of this indicates that (non-fishing) hunting is very much a minority pursuit.

Finch et al (2014), in a paper which rather breathlessly extols the virtues of hunting (for example, 'hunters must be regarded as an important part of the wildlife management community'), sought to survey Australian hunters. They did this by contacting the major hunting associations and asking their members to participate. Nobody wanted to do so unless they were anonymous – which is rather telling. Bearing in mind the severe limitations of this 'survey', it was interesting that 98% of the respondents were male. Most people justified their activities by saying they were motivated by 'pest control' and 'hunting for meat'. This would be laughable in another context; the survey did not actually ask whether those surveyed got a kick out of killing animals. Moreover, this purportedly scientific paper said nothing about animal welfare, and made no attempt to discuss its findings, other than to say that hunters spent a lot of money. The conclusion was that hunters could 'become a valuable resource to wildlife managers in this country', without supporting evidence.

Franklin (2007b) also surveyed people to find out which activities involving animals they approved or disapproved of. Thirty percent of those surveyed agreed with the proposition that hunting was an extension of natural processes that take place in the wild and was therefore acceptable. So hunting *per se* is not universally approved of, but is acceptable to a significant minority. However, 68% of people thought that it was acceptable to hunt feral animals (such as pigs) that degraded the environment; 71% of those surveyed thought the opposite about hunting native animals. So there was a dichotomy between attitudes to hunting 'pests' and attitudes to hunting native animals. I don't think these results are inconsistent with the idea that most disapprove of hunting. I think it is rather the case that people feel very negative about 'pest' animals. Questions were not asked about what happened when native animals became pests – as occurs, for example, when kangaroos are shot because they are supposed to be disturbing the environment of threatened plants or other animals. RSPCA Australia refers to its surveys which indicate that about 75% of people don't approve of hunting.[644] While there was a decrease in those licensed to hunt animals up to about 2008,[645] more recent figures appear to show that there has been a substantial increase in those licensed to kill animals. For example, in Victoria, the Game Management Authority figures show that licences to kill duck, quail and deer totalled about 48,000 in 2016, up from about 30,000 in 2009. Unsurprisingly, nearly 97% of those licensed to kill animals were males.[646]

Hunting is nominally regulated in Australia. There is a scale of regulatory strength, ranging from the almost non-existent (if the animal is considered a pest, such as a wild rabbit, pig or any other feral animal), through to the animals which society says must be protected because they are threatened with extinction. Thiriet (2009) points out that even 'threatened' animals are not protected *per se*; rather the species is protected; the practical upshot is that the welfare of an individual animal is not the issue. But in all jurisdictions, the generality is killing for fun is permitted. So, for example, 'recreational' duck hunting is permitted in South Australia, Tasmania, Victoria and the Northern Territory during open seasons, but not otherwise. Hunters are not permitted to shoot certain species and are required to pass a Waterfowl Identification Test in an attempt to ensure they don't shoot the wrong ducks. Even so (and as you would expect) there have been many instances of protected and endangered species of ducks being shot.[647] Other species which are hunted include buffaloes, camels, cats, deer,

---

[644] www.rspca.org.au/media-centre/news/2016/four-corners'-"paying-kill"-horror-show

[645] Thiriet (2009).

[646] Game Management Authority *Game Licence Statistics Summary Report 2016*.

[647] kb.rspca.org.au/What-happens-during-duck-and-quail-shooting-and-where-does-this-occur_530.html

foxes, goats, hares, pheasants, possums, pigs, rabbits, rams, geese, kangaroos, wallabies and quail. Most hunting involves shooting. Some hunters use bows and arrows. The latter is completely indefensible, as it cannot by any measure be regarded as humane. Shooting using firearms is potentially more humane, but cannot be justified morally, regardless. Likewise it is fantasy to imagine that hunting using dogs will result in anything other than the dogs bringing down the prey and causing substantial pain and damage.

Psychologist Eleonora Gullone's view, having considered the relevant literature, is that recreational hunting clearly fits within the definition of intentional cruelty; that is, behaviour performed proactively and repeatedly by an individual with the deliberate intention of causing harm to a victim with the understanding that the victim is motivated to avoid that harm. She regards recreational hunting as a demonstration of compromised empathy and compassion. She also notes that young people are at particular risk where cruel and aggressive behaviours are regarded as normal, or described as 'recreational' or 'fun'.[648] Gullone is of the view that children who witness or participate in violence and cruelty, such as hunting, are likelier to themselves become abusers. She says 'it is very bad policy to encourage children to hunt' and therefore 'it is incumbent on any responsible government to ban the activity'. I agree.

Unsurprisingly, surveys show that men who approve of hunting rate more highly than women on psychological aggression scores.[649] It will also not come as a surprise that people who engage in hunting have significantly less concern for animal welfare..[650]

Gullone (2015) points to the associations between violence, animal cruelty and participation in hunting. Those who said they hunted were about twice as likely to engage in violence towards animals as non-

---

[648] Gullone (2015).
[649] Wilson and Peden (2015).
[650] Cornish (2016).

hunters. There was a similar likelihood hunters had damaged or destroyed someone's property in their youth.

The next vexed issue under the heading of 'hunting' is fishing. Franklin (2007a) also found that a very large number of people said they went fishing. A survey carried out recently in New Zealand found that over 60% of those interviewed did not disapprove of fishing. Fishing for 'sport' or leisure is undoubtedly popular. Some have said it has '...developed into a prosperous industry providing immense benefit to society and economy'.[651] I'm not sure I would go that far.

So far as fishing is concerned, it seems quite likely that some people may release fish after they have been caught. There are indications catch and release does not result in significant mortality.[652] However, one Australian study did find such fish suffered significant fin damage and barotrauma, although the authors felt these were related to handling, so could be improved with education.[653] Some studies have found improvements can be achieved with instruction about, for example, humane killing methods.[654] There is a long way to go before anything will improve regarding fishing. Unfortunately, it really is an unassailable part of the country's psyche, so progress will be by minuscule steps, if at all.

The overall conclusion is that hunting with guns and other weapons is regulated in a desultory and superficial manner. The hunting lobby has more or less got what it wants, particularly as at the political level, it has forged an alliance with the fishing lobby (and claims to be aligned to farmers' interests). This has given the resultant Shooters, Fishers and Farmers Party an enormous amount of leverage, particularly where the major parties are unable to garner enough votes in their own rights to govern. The deals which have emerged, as a consequence, have often

---

[651] Cooke and Sneddon (2006).
[652] Ferter et al. (2017).
[653] Dowling et al. (2010).
[654] Diggles (2016).

bordered on the bizarre. One example is the approval by the New South Wales government of pest shooting by 'volunteers' in national parks.[655]

The end result is that hunting in general and fishing in particular is unlikely to be effectively controlled by governments, regardless of the serious animal welfare issues involved. This is just a further example of the long road ahead for those concerned about animal welfare.

## Commercial Hunting

There is no doubt that killing of kangaroos for meat is the largest terrestrial commercial hunting activity in Australia.[656] It goes on, under licence, in New South Wales, Queensland, South Australia and Western Australia. There is a commercial wallaby-killing industry in Tasmania. This practice is governed by 'management plans' in each jurisdiction, which are also relevant to kangaroo killing for meat intended for export.[657] The ostensible justification of kangaroo killing is to control populations, in order to prevent damage to farmers' crops. Thus, the extent of the killing is governed by quotas, which are set according to population surveys. It seems likely that the number of kangaroos killed is declining, probably because of decreasing populations and thereby increasing difficulty for shooters to make a profit. For example, in Queensland, the 2017 figures show that a total of about 331,000 were killed, and that this was about 2-15% of the quotas issued (depending on which region).[658] In New South Wales, the 2016 quotas were just

---

[655] see www.environment.nsw.gov.au/questions/licence-hunt-national-park
[656] The website of THINKK, which is an organisation dedicated to researching issues in and around kangaroo killing, is a rich source of materials: www.thinkkangaroos.uts.edu.au.
[657] see *Export Control (Wild Game Meat and Wild Game Meat Products) Orders 2010* (Cth).
[658] https://www.qld.gov.au/environment/plants-animals/wildlife-permits/macropods-qld.

over 2.5 million (against an estimated population of 17.5 million), and the number of kangaroos killed was about 200,000.[659]

All kangaroo killing licences require compliance with the *National Code of Practice for the Humane Shooting of Kangaroos and Wallabies for Commercial Purposes*.[660] This is another one of those fantasy documents. Its aim is said to be to achieve a 'sudden and humane death'. That is not to say that a commercial shooter doesn't want that to happen, because it is clear that someone who is out in the bush in the middle of the night (which is when this goes on) trying to make money out of killing kangaroos and wallabies does not want to waste time or effort wounding animals which then escape. A competent commercial killer wants to kill animals quickly. But nonsense about only shooting animals in the brain, locating wounded animals and killing them, and killing young at foot or pouch young is just that; nonsense. The 'methodology' for disposing of the very young animals involves braining them on something hard, like the bullbar of a ute. The likelier scenario is they just get left to die – but how would you ever know?

The kangaroo killing industry is a particularly brutal, dirty and unseemly business. It goes on in the bush, usually at night, and is virtually unregulated. Given that it seems as if kangaroo populations are on the way down, it seems hard to justify this commercially marginal and very likely cruel activity.

---

[659] NSW Commercial kangaroo harvest management plan 2017-21; 2017 Quota Report.
[660] National Resource Management Ministerial Council (2008).

## Chapter 11  Consumer pressure

Rachel Carson (author of *A Silent Spring*, the seminal book on environmentalism which engendered an entire influential movement) wrote a forward to Ruth Harrison's *Animal Machines*. She said about the book 'I hope it will spark a consumers' revolt of such proportions that this vast new agricultural industry will be forced to mend its ways'. Has this happened?

Consumers are becoming increasingly concerned about the food they eat, and in particular the welfare of the animals it comes from. The food industry, primarily retailers and restaurant chains (less so the producers) are starting to respond to this shift by offering high welfare products. This reflects a trend which is gathering pace in the Western world.[661] However, there is good evidence that most members of the public have little understanding of the processes involved in growing and killing animals for food.[662] Older people have less concern, and women are consistently more concerned about animal welfare than men.

Interestingly, some of this pressure has come from overseas. Responding to pressure from its customers about the use of mulesing, prestigious Italian clothing manufacture Ermenegildo Zegna decided in 2009 to cancel its award for high quality wool sourced from Australia and New Zealand. The award was reinstated in 2010, but only for wool from non-mulesed sheep. At the moment, Zegna's awards include wool from mulesed sheep which have been given pain relief.[663] In similar vein, international clothing retailer H&M has instigated a policy that wool originated from Australia must not come from mulesed sheep.[664]

---

[661] Maloni and Brown (2006).

[662] Cornish et al. (2016).

[663] Australian Woolgrowers' Association (April 2017) *Zegna's wool growing pains*; see also www.zegna.com.au/au-en/editorial/fabrics/ermenegildo-zegna-wool-award.html.

[664] H&M *Animal Welfare Policy* www.sustainability.hm.com/en/sustainability/download-

Recent reports indicate that non-mulesed superfine wool commands a premium price from Italian buyers.[665]

It has often been said that consumers, while being concerned about poor animal welfare are unwilling to pay to improve it. This sort of line is run repeatedly in assessments carried out by economic consultants for government, under the heading of 'willingness to pay'.[666] I think the events of the last couple of decades have shown that consumers are indeed willing to pay. Jed Goodfellow (2015) reviews studies of consumer attitudes which confirm that consumers are in fact willing to pay more for good animal welfare when purchasing animal-derived products. Broom (2011) pointed out that the proportion of French consumers who buy products such as chicken meat only on price is thought to have dropped to 25%. This was by reference to the French 'Label Rouge' scheme, which uses slower growing meat chickens which do not experience the dreadful health problems associated with the common strains used by the industry. The Productivity Commission's 2017 report on *Regulation of Australian Agriculture* cites evidence that 'consumers assign a positive value to increased animal welfare'.

While surveys of intentions and reported changes in purchasing behaviour can be informative, the real question is whether people are changing what they buy because of animal welfare concerns, and whether they are prepared to pay more. Consumers are very obviously prepared to pay more for free range products, particularly eggs, otherwise there would not be so many examples of producers falsely labelling eggs as 'free range' when they are in fact from battery hens. The Australian Consumer and Competition Commission has successfully

---

resources/policies/policies/animal-welfare-policy.html. Note this policy includes that by the end of 2017, its sources should comply with requirements based on the Five Freedoms.

[665] https://www.sheepcentral.com/italian-processors-pay-400-cent-plus-premiums-for-non-mulesed-superfine-wool.

[666] Older studies indicated that people's good intentions were unlikely to manifest as a willingess to pay for improved animal welfare. See Taylor and Signal (2009).

prosecuted several producers under the Australian Consumer Law for these misleading practices.[667] Consumers who buy free range eggs may also (wrongly) assume that the eggs are tastier and more nutritious; indeed this may be a stronger motivator for some than concern for animal welfare.[668] Ironically, concern for the quality of food, rather than solely animal welfare, was a significant driver of improvements in the early 1800s (although it must be said that food animals in those days probably were in a shocking state, with disease and poor health the norm).[669]

But it should be remembered that not all consumers are able to afford the luxury of having moral standards which will increase the cost of their food choices. Webster (1994) has rightly said that 'food prices for all should not be distorted by welfare standards prescribed by a vocal and affluent minority'. But this should all be tempered by asking whether the increased expenditure involved in buying improved-welfare products is actually that significant, in the scale of things.

The recent figures from Australian Egg Corporation Limited (2016) on egg production show that for the first time, free range grocery egg sales (by value) have overtaken sales of eggs produced in all other housing systems, including battery cages. The cost of free range eggs averaged $5.45 per dozen, compared to $3.22 per dozen for cage eggs. Barn-laid eggs sold for $4.68 per dozen. This clearly shows that consumers' views, as shown in surveys, are translated into reality when making purchasing decisions. Likewise there has been growth in purchasing higher welfare chicken meat, such as those sold under RSPCA Australia's Approved Farming Scheme.[670] Note, however, that if all eggs (including those going to the food service industry) are taken into account, cage layer

---

[667] *ACCC v Pirovic Enterprises Pty Ltd (No 2)* [2014] FCA 1028; *ACCC v RL Adams Pty Ltd* [2015] FCA 1016; *ACCC v Derodi Pty Ltd* [2016] FCA 365; *ACCC v Snowdale Holdings Pty Ltd* [2016] FCA 541.
[668] Bray and Ankeny (2017).
[669] Kean (1998).
[670] see Goodfellow (2015).

farming still constitutes 68% of total egg production.[671] The significance of this is that consumers still need to be educated regarding the source of eggs which goes into cakes, biscuits, prepared meals and the like.

When surveyed, consumers say that their main reasons for buying 'free range' eggs is that chickens are able to move about freely and have access to the outdoors.[672] It has been said that a maximum stocking density of 1 hen per square metre is regarded as acceptable to only 2 per cent of consumers.[673] But it is quite clear that a very significant proportion of consumers has no idea about what keeping egg-laying chickens in a 'free range' environment really means. There tends to be an unjustified reliance on stocking density as the parameter on which to base a judgement.

As mentioned in Chapter 4, consumer affairs ministers from the various Australian jurisdictions have acted to seek to provide some certainty regarding the definition of 'free range' eggs, at least so far as stocking density of the outside range is concerned. There is now an information standard made under the Australian Consumer Law to the effect that 'free range' means a maximum stocking density of 10,000 hens per hectare (that is, 1 hen per square metre).[674]

There is every reason to acknowledge that animal welfare, rather than being 'intangible' (that is, derived from ethics and moral values) and a 'public good', actually has a financial value.[675] Producers would do well to take note of this.

---

[671] RSPCA Australia (2016).
[672] Productivity Commission (2017).
[673] Choice, quoted in Productivity Commission (2017).
[674] *Australian Consumer Law (Free Range Egg Labelling) Information Standard 2017* (Cth). This also requires that hens have meaningful and regular access to an outdoor range during daylight hours and are able to roam and forage on the range.
[675] Dawkins (2017b).

Driven by concerns expressed by consumers, major players in the food industry have started a push towards 'welfare friendly' products. This is of particular importance, given the enormous power of food retailers.[676] These shifts reflect a recognition by at least some major corporate concerns of the need to behave ethically in their business practices; many (but not the majority) such companies publish animal welfare policies and objectives.[677] Of course, it is one thing having policies and so on; it is another thing entirely whether this improves the lives of animals. In Australia, serious public concern for the welfare of intensively farmed animals has in recent years resulted in major supermarket chain Coles stopping the sale of its own brand eggs from caged chickens, or pork from facilities where pregnant pigs are kept in small sow stalls. Food retailer Woolworths has partly followed suit regarding its own label products. In like vein, major fast food chain McDonald's has committed to use only eggs from cage free facilities by 2017. There are media reports that burger restaurant chain Hungry Jack's has already transitioned to using eggs from cage-free sources.[678]

It has often been said that much criticism of agricultural practices might frequently be based on a poor understanding of conditions on farms.[679] While there is much that is positive about the effects of consumer pressure, the problem is that public opinion is often fragmented and ambiguous, being influenced by a range of elements which means the views held are not necessarily rational or based on facts.[680] That range of elements can include factors such as the level of knowledge and understanding, personal preferences and biases, and most importantly, the relative importance of a particular animal welfare issue compared to other issues of concern to members of the public.[681] These things, perhaps the most important of which will be factors relating to personal

---

[676] See Thompson et al. (2007).
[677] see Sullivan (2017).
[678] see RSPCA Australia (2016).
[679] Weary et al. (2016).
[680] See Bloom (2008); Degeling and Johnson (2015).
[681] Chen (2016); Timoshanko (2015).

wealth and wellbeing, will probably trump concerns about animal welfare. Southwell et al. (2006) found that a sample of 1,000 Australians rated health, inflation, family relationships, tax reform, education, terrorism, the environment and unemployment as more important [682]

The online survey conducted in 2013 by Humane Research Council indicated that many persons (over 60%) claimed to have bought products labelled 'free range' or the equivalent. Chen (2016) views these figures as somewhat optimistic – he thinks people will say they prefer humane products, but when it comes to buying food or other animal-based commodities, they will be heavily influenced by price, availability and other factors. Another obvious concern relates to what is on the product label. For a label like 'free range' to mean something, there has to be a standard which can be enforced. The difficulty with that is again that the consumer may not necessarily have a sufficiently deep understanding of what an animal welfare friendly term may in fact mean. Thus, when the egg industry says, for example, it has surveyed people and they think chickens are likely to be content with having one square metre of space each on a range, what that does not say is whether the same people would be equally happy knowing that those birds are housed in sheds containing 25,000 birds or more. The consumer just does not have sufficient knowledge of the system, and the industry is unlikely to bare its soul without having to. As Geoff Bloom has said, labelling is 'a blunt and ineffective instrument for regulating animal welfare'.[683]

Even accepting that, there has been increasing use of application of standards by non-government agencies, which in effect endorse products produced in a particular way. RSPCA Australia leads the way in this regard. Attempts by industry to impose voluntary codes must be viewed with suspicion; their track record in this regard concerning

---

[682] cited in Chen (2016).
[683] Bloom (2008).

stopping mulesing of lambs and keeping pregnant pigs in sow stalls has not been good.

Another important point is that relying on markets to adequately protect animal welfare is unlikely to be satisfactory because economic values express only what each market participant is willing to pay in exchange for something else. The final word, therefore, is that social and ethical values must be dealt with by governments, and I think that is what voters expect.[684]

---

[684] See Bloom (2008).

# Chapter 12  Companion animals

My personal view, which will be regarded by many as extreme, is that keeping companion animals, which necessarily involves restricting their freedom and may involve surgical mutilations and other interventions, could be said to not be in the best interests of the animals concerned. Keeping pets is not a trivial matter; poor training, feeding, restraint or lack of treatment are some examples of obvious failures of proper care and can cause serious difficulties for the animal.

Adrian Franklin (2007a) reported that nearly 70% of Australians kept at least one animal on their property; most of these were companion animal species. Dogs were most popular, followed by cats, birds, fish and rabbits. This survey also indicated a move away from largely keeping companion animals outside. Franklin believes that the primary motivation of many Australians for keeping companion animals is because of loneliness. Crucially, he notes that most Australians regard their companion animals as family members. Today, two thirds of households regard their cats or dogs as part of the family.[685] Unsurprisingly, people who have had or do have a companion animal are likelier to be concerned about animal welfare in general.[686]

Recent information[687] indicates that 38% of Australian households have at least one dog; the total estimated dog population is 4.8 million. Of these, half are pure breeds and more than a third of dogs are acquired through a breeder. Only 16% come from animal shelters, although this is slightly more than those sourced from pet shops. Twenty percent of dogs are exclusively kept outdoors; more dogs (27%) are kept outdoors in regional areas. One troubling statistic is that 15% of all dogs are kept exclusively at home. Seventy eight percent of dogs are desexed.

Cats are present in 29% of Australian households; the estimated population is 3.9 million. A quarter of cats are acquired through animal

---

[685] Animal Medicines Australia (2016) *Pet ownership in Australia*.
[686] Cornish et al. (2014).
[687] Animal Medicines Australia (2016) *Pet ownership in Australia*.

shelters. Fifteen percent of people say their cats are strays which they have adopted. Eighty nine percent of cats are desexed.

Eighty three percent of dogs are microchipped, while 72% of cats are microchipped. Microchipping of dogs and cats is compulsory in New South Wales, Victoria, Queensland, ACT and Western Australia.[688] There is a particular issue with pet cats, in that they are usually allowed to roam outside the home. This can result in nuisance to neighbours, as well as risks to the welfare of the cats themselves; this can come from being struck by vehicles or from fighting with other cats.[689] My personal view, likely to be very unpopular with some, is that cats should not be allowed to roam freely, for these reasons.

Twelve percent of households keep fish (of which there are about 8.7 million; this is a decrease of just over 20% since 2013).

Those involved with companion animal welfare regularly express concern over the level of killing of unwanted and stray animals. There is no doubt this is a major issue. Although it is obviously preferable for people to get 'rescue' animals as companions, rather than buying them from breeders, pet shops and so on, this may not be suitable or appropriate for many. Some rescue dogs and cats may just be impossible for people to deal with. The inevitable result must be that they will have to be killed. RSPCA Australia reports that over the three years since it previously reported, both the number and proportion of animals euthanased by RPSCAs has declined; from just under 50,000 in 2011-12 to about 40,300 in 2014-15.

The issue with abandoned and unwanted animals is really one of lack of education. People should be made aware that taking on a pet is a huge responsibility and they should know about all the potential problems.

---

[688] *Companion Animal Act 1998* (NSW); *Domestic Animals Act 1994* (Vic); *Animal Management (Cats and Dogs) Act 2008* (Qld); *Companion Animals Act 1998* (ACT); *Dog Act 1976* (WA); *Cat Act 2011* (WA).
[689] Hall et al. (2016).

Most importantly, they should know that it is an ongoing and long-lasting commitment. Governments should provide education, or at least be supporting animal welfare organisations in doing that. One of the triggers for abandonment of animals is the difficulty that tenants have in finding rental accommodation which allows them to keep pets. It may be that things will improve in this regard in Victoria, where the government has announced that the *Residential Tenancies Act* will be revised to give tenants a right to keep a pet.[690]

The majority of pet owners are female, younger, employed, quite well off financially, and own their own home. Just under half are from a non-English-speaking background. An interesting statistic is that for both dogs and cats. most are acquired cost-free or for very little cost.

There are data showing that keepers of companion animals spend about $8 billion each year on their pets.[691] The general public has much more interest in issues relating to companion animals than to other animals (including farm animals). This is reflected in media reporting of matters concerning animals, which prior to the live export scandal of 2011 was largely about cruelty to cats and dogs, having a crime emphasis.[692]

The association between dogs and humans is at least 12,000 years old.[693] That particular association may to some degree be dependent on members of the one species regarding the member of the other species as being a member of their pack or tribe. This would not necessarily be so for many species. Over the years of this association, dogs have been bred to have 'desirable' features (usually appearance-related), including size, face type, length of leg, running speed, and so on. This has been done while disregarding the negative genetic consequences of

---

[690] 'Victorian tenants given right to have a pet under sweeping changes to rental laws.' ABC News, 8 October 2017. www.abc.net.au/news/2017-10-08/victorian-tenants-allowed-pets-in-rental-properties/9027000.
[691] White (2016).
[692] Chen (2012).
[693] Broom and Fraser (2007).

the inbreeding, resulting in many dogs having hearing disorders, hyperexcitability, hip dysplasia, tendency to seizures, ingrowing eyelashes, and many other complaints which clearly result in bad welfare.[694] Dogs are routinely mutilated to make them easier to keep and handle; the most widespread mutilations are castration of males and spaying of females. These mutilations result in major behavioural changes, and could thereby be said to cause poor welfare; however, it is also arguable that the consequent increase in freedom offsets this to some extent. One major problem with dogs kept in a restricted environment for any length of time is separation anxiety.[695] This may be ameliorated to some extent by keeping more than one dog.[696]

Humans and cats have associated for at least 9,500 years. Broom and Fraser (2007) are of the view that, production of particular cat breeds over the years has often been associated with the selection of attributes which result in poor welfare. They give examples of bad attributes, including excessively nervous tendencies, high levels of aggression and predisposition to serious diseases. As with dogs, castration and spaying of cats is commonly practised and is necessarily associated with behavioural changes. The tendency to allow cats to roam freely outside the home environment is associated with many problems. As mentioned, there is a risk they will suffer injury or be killed by motor vehicles; in the rural environment, there is a risk they will be shot. Farmers, in my experience, are quite obsessed with the idea that feral cats are a 'bad thing' and when they see a cat and shoot it, they are unconcerned whether or not it may be someone's pet.

Most who study the area would agree that there are real physiological and psychological benefits to owners of companion animals. These result from the care and compassion associated with keeping companion animals, and can be seen in positive effects on persons

---

[694] Broom and Fraser (2007).
[695] see Webster (2005).
[696] Broom and Fraser (2007).

suffering depression, who are socially isolated, or who are anxious.[697] Melson (2003)[698] has described the positive effects on child development of the presence of a companion animal during a child's upbringing.

Enforcement of the animal welfare and cruelty law relating to companion animals is usually outsourced by state and territory governments to RSPCAs.[699] White (2016) expresses the view that the way in which the law about companion animals is framed emphasises values other than just those governed by market efficiency or economics. He also makes the point (quoting Sunstein) that the property status of companion animals may not serve as too much of a brake on the protection offered to them by the law, as 'those who have bought their dog do not think that they own a "thing"'. However, he rightly points to problems with 'puppy farms' and bad breeding practices which may be exacerbated by the property status of pets.

The law relating to companion animals (essentially cats and dogs)[700] reflects the schizophrenia in this country concerning those animals. Much of what those acts seek to achieve (for example registration of dogs, their identification; compulsory microchipping and so on) is laudable; but equally, a lot of what has ended up in legislation represents victimisation, dressed up as a requirement for good management. For example, in New South Wales it is an offence for a person who is in charge of a dog in a public place (unless the area is a declared 'off-leash area') if the dog is not on a lead (although as one would expect, this does not apply to farmers). Farmers also have *carte blanche* to kill dogs and cats on their land, even if those animals are doing nothing. Dogs and cats can be seized if they are a 'nuisance'. But a far more insidious and worrying trend is the idea that there are

---

[697] Westbury et al. (2011).

[698] Child development and the human-companion animal bond. *American Behavioral Scientist* 47, 31-39.

[699] see White (2016).

[700] eg *Companion Animals Act 1998* (NSW); *Domestic Animals Act 1994* (Vic);

'dangerous' or 'menacing' dogs, or worse still, breeds of dogs,[701] which can be subjected to all sorts of intervention, including killing them. This sort of legislation ignores the fact that much of the problem with dogs arises because of the failure of their owners. For example, a dog which is allowed to interact with young children while not being under effective control may well attack those children. This is entirely to be expected, particularly in a family environment. The fact is that dog owners have a huge responsibility to ensure their animals are under control, and often fail. Any dog can be dangerous if it is not adequately trained and controlled. Moreover, anti-dangerous dog legislation often encourages those responsible for enforcing it (principally council employees) to behave in a draconian manner.

Another important issue concerning laws relating to companion animals (cats and dogs) is that local authorities are expected to do a lot of the heavy lifting when it comes to issues like registration, dealing with stray animals and so on. It is apparent that this creates a significant resource problem for local authorities. For example, the recent proposal for a 'puppy farm' Bill in Victoria was essentially rejected by the reviewing committee for reasons which included lack of proper resourcing for local councils to enable them to carry out their enforcement tasks.[702]

Despite all this interest, what is clearly lacking in Australian law is a definition of minimum acceptable standards for keeping cats and dogs. So far as I am aware, it is still the law almost everywhere in this country that a dog can be kept on a chain or rope for most of its life, getting next to no exercise. In Tasmania a dog cannot be tethered for more than 30 minutes unless it 'shows acceptance of being tethered and is not distressed as a result' and is exercised daily (being a reasonable opportunity to exercise for at least 60 minutes in total). I note in passing that while the latter stipulation is laudable, it is unenforceable. How

---

[701] Dogs which are the subject of special provisions in legislation include pit bulls, Japanese tosa, dogo Argentino and fila Brasileiro.

[702] Legislative Council Economy and Infrastructure Committee *Inquiry into the Domestic Animals Amendment (Puppy Farms and Pet Shops) Bill 2016.*

would you ever know how frequently and for how long a dog had been exercised? Other such legislation is weak. For example, in New South Wales, it is an offence to tether an animal 'for an unreasonable length of time'.[703] What does that mean?

The issue of 'puppy farms' is one which has stirred up a fair bit of public interest. In my view, it is something of a distraction, as the real question is how dog breeders should be registered and managed *per se*. Somehow the idea has taken hold that any large dog breeding operation is suspect, and probably will be associated with bad animal welfare. RSPCA VIctoria has defined a puppy farm as 'an intensive dog breeding facility that is operated under inadequate conditions that fail to meet the dogs' behavioural, social and/or physiological needs'. That is fine – but that means, impliedly, that one can operate an intensive breeding facility under adequate conditions. And why not? The recent (failed) Victorian Bill sought to reduce the number of fertile females which could be used for breeding by a breeder to 10. Some breeders currently have up to 300 breeding females. While the Minister claimed RSPCA Victoria had arrived at the limit of 10 breeding females based on science, testimony from that organisation did not support this.[704]

My view is that if 'puppy farms' are an issue, then the answer is not restricting the size of the operations, but making sure that all pet breeding operations are properly conducted and policed. That necessarily is going to involve providing more resources, which governments will always be reluctant to do.

Cats and dogs will be kept as pets for the foreseeable future. In order to minimise the trauma to the animals, pet owners need to be educated regarding proper treatment and care of their animals. Those who cannot provide this should be prevented from keeping animals. That said, it is likely that those who dislike cats and dogs will continue to exert

---

[703] *Prevention of Cruelty to Animals Act 1979* (NSW) s10(1).
[704] Legislative Council Economy and Infrastructure Committee *Inquiry into the Domestic Animals Amendment (Puppy Farms and Pet Shops) Bill 2016.*

significant influence over laws and regulations. This aspect of the Australian schizophrenia towards animals is unlikely to change any time soon.

# Chapter 13  Wildlife and feral animals

Wildlife and feral animals must be dealt with under the same heading, as both classes of animals inhabit the same space. Moreover, many of the same biases against animals can come to apply to both categories, so when, for example, a native animal interferes with human activity, it is persecuted just as much as a feral.

Likewise when a preferred domestic animal, be it a pet (such as a cat or dog) or a farmed animal (such as a pig) crosses the line to a 'feral', it can be persecuted mercilessly, once it is no longer in the domestic domain.

A major part of the problem is the inability of Australians to accept that the countryside is irreversibly changed, and that there is no longer any such thing as 'natural'. The intervention of humanity has resulted in both the introduction of many non-native animals, which will never be eradicated or controlled, and the growth of populations of some native animals, which have benefitted from feeding on pasture and crops. For some reason, rather than grasp the reality of a hybrid Australia, so far as animals are concerned, there is a constant striving for an unattainable 'pure Australia'; this is Australian eco-nationalism.[705]

Adrian Franklin (2007a) beautifully summarises the Australian double standard about native versus introduced wildlife, and the perceived scourge of the feral animal. All of these quite odd attitudes tie in nicely with nationalistic fervour. He quotes Janet Holmes à Court (wannabe president of Australia and serial industrial-scale cattle producer and live exporter), who said:

> *'We need the smell of eucalyptus in this and the feel of red dust. We need to have the feel of swimming in the sea and all those things that make us feel so passionate about this country and love it so much – eating beef and no feral cats'.*

---

[705] see Franklin (2007a).

Difficult to keep a straight face when reading this tosh. But it unfortunately resonates with many.

Biodiversity is a fashionable concept these days. It is said to be 'the variety of all living organisms, at all levels of organisation'. In considering why biodiversity matters, a recent CSIRO book[706] on the subject refers to five primary values: economic, ecological life-support, recreation, cultural values and scientific. Of course 'economic value' must represent an anti-biodiversity value. For example, surely farming is anti-biodiversity? One cannot farm without creating a monoculture of one sort or another. But moving on from that, what those values do not mention is any reason why one should be concerned about species extinctions. I can understand, for example, why an aesthetic view might justify such concern – that is entirely valid. It's as valid as appreciating the Mona Lisa. But what seems to have happened is a complete obsession with this aspect of biodiversity and threats to it, particularly where the threat is said to be posed by feral animals or over-abundance of native animals. Those threats get the blame well ahead of every human activity which threatens species with extinction. Forget feral cats; think land clearing, think palm oil.[707]

Adrian Franklin's report of Australian attitudes to animals rather surprisingly found that a significant majority of people had a very positive view of wild animals. Many species of wild animals were encountered in people's local environment, and indeed were tolerated and fed. Again, surprisingly, less than half of those surveyed were 'anxious' about wild animals.[708]

[706] 'Biodiversity' (2014) www.publish.csiro.au/ebook/download/pdf/6967.
[707] Adrian Franklin (2007a) offers an intriguing account of Aboriginal attitudes to wild and feral animals, and the need to conserve some and exterminate others. He describes how many Aboriginal persons simply do not understand why anyone would want to do this.
[708] Franklin (2007b).

The overriding ethos regarding animals in the wild, whether feral or native, is that if they interfere with human activities, particularly farming, then they can be killed. The interference can either be by killing the farmers' animals, or eating their crops, or even (for example in the case of wombats) by digging holes. The methods used to kill these 'pests' are almost all horrendous. They are trapped, poisoned, shot, or blown up. I suggest that because much of what goes on is out of sight, there is absolutely no regard for the welfare of these unfortunate creatures. Furthermore, the obsession of farming communities with destroying anything which is perceived as interfering with profit-making is associated, I think, with an attitude which borders on the sadistic.

The obsession of the relevant authorities with killing as almost the sole means of control of feral animals or over-populous native wildlife is now being questioned. Some of these programmes have been successful in limiting predation by feral species on islands or in local fenced-off areas. But these interventions are very costly and are probably ineffective (apart from those few isolated cases) in arresting the decline of threatened fauna. Indeed, some have pointed out that they can result in a negative outcome for biodiversity.[709]

It is easy to see that as far as a farmer is concerned, the ecological status of a particular species is only looked at through the lens of profit. If an animal is large and eats the farmers' crops, or the farmers' animals, it will be hunted mercilessly. Once its numbers have declined to the point where the species is threatened, then the farmers are no longer concerned.

Australian attitudes and policy regarding wildlife are biased positively towards those (native) animals seen to be threatened with extinction. In this framework it is permissible to exterminate large numbers of members of populous native species in order to preserve those who are said to be threatened. Thus, kangaroos are the particular *bêtes noirs*

---

[709] Doherty et al. (2015a).

when it comes to the need to kill large numbers of them in order to protect animals or plants said to be 'threatened'. This raises obvious welfare concerns.[710]

In an ironic twist, while the federal government has rid itself of any involvement in looking after animal welfare, it has wholeheartedly embraced an assault on unwanted native wildlife and feral animals. In my view this is a further example of the attitudes of farmers infiltrating government of the entire country. This assault occurs through powers under the *Environment Protection and Biodiversity Conservation Act 1999*. At this point, I think it is necessary to pause and ask why biodiversity is so important. Is it because of a Noah's Ark view of wildlife, whereby those concerned have a nice warm glow because they conserve animal species? Or is it because protection of biodiversity allows humans to give vent to their seemingly overwhelming urge to exert power and control over everything in the environment? Whatever the reason, the outcome for the unfortunate 'pests' is terrible.

'Control' of over-populous wildlife, or killing of noisome pests (which can be either native wildlife or introduced species) involves various methods, all of which are cruel, in my view. To pretend they are 'humane' is to delude oneself; use of these approaches will inevitably result in bad animal welfare.[711] Poisons are frequently used. Examples are sodium fluoroacetate (1080 – a metabolic poison; think cyanide) and anticoagulants (such as brodifacoum – a commonly used rat poison, which is now used for other species such as rabbits; think bleeding to death internally); brodifacoum can take 21 days to kill, with a duration of 'sickness' of 7 days.[712] Compared to other poisons, it is probably the worst.[713]

---

[710] Fraser (2012).

[711] Littin et al. (2014).

[712] See the references in Littin et al. (2004).

[713] Littin et al. (2014).

All of these poisons kill in a way which is to some extent slow and thereby probably bad for the welfare of the target animal.[714] It is clear that those advocating the use of poisons to get rid of unwanted wildlife or feral animals run the risk of losing public approval if the methods they use are perceived as cruel.[715]

Fluoroacetate (1080) has been the subject of concern, as it probably produces many unpleasant effects before animals succumb. The evidence of Littin et al. (2009) in possums was that the animals showed lack of coordination about 3 hours after dosing, with some exhibiting spasms and tremors, or seizures. Animals receiving sublethal doses had abnormal postures, lack of coordination, retching, and cessation of grooming and activity. The authors noted the animals were probably unconscious during the seizures, but that leaving seizures aside, the animals given lethal doses were probably conscious for over 9 hours before death. They concluded it was 'undesirable' for animal welfare. Twigg and Parker (2010) have argued that 1080 is in fact humane, because there is a lag before any effects are observed and because 1080 impairs neurological functioning, there is a good chance the poisoned animals are not experiencing pain.[716] To support this, they refer to effects on neuronal acetylcholine and glutamate, which are neurotransmitters, although they provide no support for their assertion beyond this bald statement. Having spent most of my time as a scientist working on acetylcholine systems, I think I can safely say that this logic is suspect. If they claim that the animals are not feeling pain or distress in response to the poison, they must present evidence that is the case. Otherwise the animals must be given the benefit of the doubt.

It is possible that 'Feratox', a form of pelletised cyanide, may be a more humane alternative than 1080, as (at least in wallabies) the time to unconsciousness is significantly shorter than 1080, being about 14

---

[714] Beausoleil et al. (2016).
[715] Littin et al. (2004).
[716] Twigg and Parker (2010).

minutes on average.[717] But all of this push for 'humane' poisons surely misses the point that animals which receive a less than lethal dose will nevertheless suffer very unpleasant symptoms. This can hardly be said to be good welfare.

Trapping is widely used as a tool to dispose of unwanted wildlife and feral animals. It has obvious negative consequences for welfare, particularly where leghold traps are used. Cage-type traps are preferable.[718]

## Feral animals

Part of the process of colonisation of Australia by European settlers involved domestic animals being shipped to Australia, either as food sources, or as sources of power (motive and otherwise), or to accommodate the taste of the gentry for hunting things. Indeed Franklin (2007a) presents a compelling argument that this activity was part of the British attempt to remodel Australia in the likeness of Britain. Many of those introduced animals were subsequently left to their own devices, or escaped. This formed the bases of the starter populations of Australia's feral animals. They don't qualify for the sort of feelgood sentiment that is applied to native animals. And because they are not owned by anybody, very few people have an interest in their welfare. They include foxes, cats, dogs, rabbits, goats, horses, deer, camels, pigs, donkeys, cane toads, buffalo and some unfortunate species of fish (such as the carp).

Feral animals which are predators, such as the cat or fox, have been said to contribute to the extinction of many species; it is thought 20 Australian mammal species have been lost by fox and cat predation.[719]

Australian farmers, and to some extent members of the public, have a loathing of feral animals. Concern for animal welfare disappears when

---

[717] Eason et al. (2010).
[718] Littin et al. (2014).
[719] Doherty and Ritchie (2017).

the subject of ire is a 'feral'. In this regard, the farmers have convinced the general community that anything which threatens (or is imagined to threaten) their livelihoods by killing farm animals can be destroyed in any way, no matter how cruelly. Or rather, we will kill them, or attempt to kill them, and pretend we are doing it humanely.

Adrian Franklin (2007a) makes the interesting point that indigenous Australians probably have a very different view. For example, Aborigines in northern Australia have a very positive attitude towards feral buffalo and cats.

The idea that feral predators, such as cats and foxes, are the sole reason for threats to some native species is naive. The ultimate impact of these predators is but one factor; other factors, which are human-controlled can be additive or synergistic.[720] The focus on the role of feral predators as a sole cause of threats to other species ignores, for example, the effect of land clearing, which is a characteristic of the modern Australian rural scene. Land clearing obviously removes natural habitat and replaces it, usually with agricultural development. This environment may enhance its suitability for introduced predators. For example, cleared land and linear features such as roads act as movement pathways and hunting areas. The occurrence of foxes and cats is positively associated with these environments. Likewise burning of areas to reduce fuel load, and thereby reduce bushfire intensity, can dramatically enhance predation effectiveness. Grazing by herbivores (particularly cows and sheep) removes vegetation cover and can expose prey to their predators. For example, feral cats in northern Australia have been found to prefer hunting in recently grazed or burned areas. Persecuting top predators, such as dingoes, can result in higher cat and fox activity. The bottom line is that attempting to kill ferals is doomed to failure and inflicts unimaginable cruelty. A holistic view of the

---

[720] Doherty et al., (2015).

environment which takes all these different factors into account, is surely the way forward.[721]

There may be large numbers of feral cats in Australia; estimates go as high as 63 million. The perceived wisdom is that feral cats are implicated in most recent mammal extinctions and continue to threaten native species.[722] Feral cats are listed as a 'key threat' to biodiversity under the *Environment Protection and Biodiversity Conservation Act 1999* (Cth). Studies have shown that, across Australia, feral cats kill about 400 vertebrate species, being 123 birds, 157 reptiles, 58 marsupials, 27 rodents, 5 bats, 21 frogs and 9 exotic mammals. Of these, there are published accounts of cat predation on 28 species that are listed as from 'near threatened' (12) to 'critically endangered'. However, a recent detailed analysis of studies of the diet of feral cats in Australia showed that rabbits are often the staple prey.[723] When fewer rabbits are available, feral cats are able to switch to other prey, such as rodents and smaller mammals. Obviously, eradicating rabbits can have the result that feral cats will switch from eating rabbits to eating something felt to be requiring conservation.

Feral cats are also probably responsible for many outbreaks of infection with toxoplasmosis, a disease which is devastating for many species of native wildlife, such as wombats.[724]

Cats are difficult to control as they tend not to consume poison baits, or enter traps when live prey are available.[725] Where attempts have been made to control cat populations in 'open' areas (ie, other than on small islands or fenced-off areas), paradoxically, feral cat numbers have been seen to increase after culling programmes, and in any case come back to pre-cull levels after the killing ceases. This happens because culling

---

[721] Doherty et al. (2017).
[722] Legge et al. (2017).
[723] Doherty et al. (2015b).
[724] Fancourt and Jackson (2014).
[725] Read et al. (2015).

removes dominant resident cats, allowing influx of younger or previously subordinate individuals from surrounding areas.[726] There is an obsession with the idea that feral cats can be eradicated in Australia. This is an impossible dream. If the impact of feral cat populations are to be managed, this must involve a targetted approach, designed specifically to address particular problems. For example, a locus of a particular threatened species may have cats excluded by fencing. What will not work is an unthinking and indiscriminate cull.[727]

The fiasco of the imaginary Tasmanian fox illustrates well how obsession can overtake reason where feral animals are concerned. For more than 15 years there was a great debate about whether foxes were present in Tasmania. Even though there was no definitive evidence, in 2001 the Tasmanian government put in place a Fox Eradication Program, ultimately costing taxpayers in excess of $50 million. This program included spreading the poison 1080 over more than a million hectares. The wider animal welfare implications of this distribution of poison are obvious, although there was never any attempt to quantify the consequences of this exercise on other animals. An independent group of international scientists has now carried out studies including examining detection and patterns of 'fox positive' scats, using molecular techniques, analysis of reliability of anecdotal sightings and a review of the efficacy of the 1080 baiting strategy. Even though there were over 3,000 anecdotal reports of fox sightings, none of these were corroborated with physical data. However, they were correlated with the intensity of media reports.[728] The attribution of scats to foxes was based on polymerase chain reaction (PCR) analysis to detect fox DNA. However, this technique is notoriously inaccurate where the 'primer' DNA sequence is able to provide amplifying signals to false positive sequences from DNA in other species. Goncalves et al. (2014) reported that strong amplifications were obtained from the relevant 'primer'

[726] Lazenby et al. (2015); Doherty and Ritchie (2017).
[727] Doherty et al. (2016).
[728] Layton-Bennett (2014).

exposed to DNA from other species which might be expected to be present in scats from predators such as quolls and Tasmanian devils.

Tasmania was home to another load of environmental nonsense involving pests a few years ago. Sub-Antarctic Macquarie Island, which has sainted conservation status, had a population of feral cats (probably no more than 200), which were said to be threatening some species of birds. So, between 1985 and 2000 the feral cats were got rid of, largely by hunting with dogs. There was a subsequent population explosion of rabbits, probably resulting from the removal of their peak predator, the feral cat. The net result was that the growth in the rabbit population started to threaten the ecosystem of the island, primarily because of burrowing.[729] To put this right, the 'eradication specialists' dumped 200 tonnes of the anticoagulant toxin brodifacoum by aerial distribution over most of the island. However, this sledgehammer did not crack the nut (seemingly due to 'adverse weather conditions'), requiring the spread of Rabbit Haemorrhagic Virus to complete the task. The proponents of this exercise claim it is a resounding success based on 'preliminary empirical and anecdotal evidence';[730] this is therefore a baseless conclusion. Clearly there is a lesson to be learned – don't interfere with an ecosystem unless you understand all the consequences.[731] In an interesting article on this debacle in *The Quadrant*, John Reid concluded:

> *'There seems to be this puritanical impulse among environmental types to restore the world, or parts of it, to some imagined, stable, pre-industrial glory, where every prospect pleases and only man is vile. There is a life-hating, totalitarian streak about this mindset, a failure to accept the world as it is, warts and all. The ruthless extermination of Macquarie Island's...cats and rabbits in*

---

[729] Bergstrom et al. (2009).
[730] Springer (2016).
[731] See Doherty and Ritchie (2017).

*the name of science stands as a testament to the treachery of good
intentions – good intentions poorly thought through'.*[732]

## Wildlife

To be classified as a native wild animal in Australia is good fortune for
those creatures involved. You become identified with Australianness,
and most of the time people will go out of their way to protect you.
There will be laws passed to do this. National parks will be established
to provide environment. Scientists and politicians will proclaim your
value. You will be cuddled by visiting dignitaries. It is likely (if you are
cute) you may become an icon of the country and your symbol will
appear on coins, flags, coats of arms, and the tails of aeroplanes. This is
what Adrian Franklin describes as part of the 'cultural taxonomy of
Australian animals'.[733] None of which makes any logical sense.

Wild animals are in an odd position. Unlike farm animals, companion
animals and so on, they are not owned by anybody. That immediately
raises the question of who is responsible for the welfare of wild animals.
Some are of the view that the moral standing of wild animals is
determined by their wild nature. As a consequence, there is a view that
wild animals should not be interfered with.[734] If one takes the view that
natural behaviours are important to animals, and allowing them to
express natural behaviours is good for welfare, then it is apparent that
animals living in the wild exemplify this state. However, it is also true
that animals in the wild can experience significant suffering and states
of negative affect.[735] Obviously, they can suffer from lack of water or
food, they can be caught by predators, and so on.[736]

Humanity is the greatest threat to wildlife. Habitats for wild animals are
threatened    worldwide    by    fragmentation,    contamination    and

---

[732] Reid (2012).
[733] Franklin (2007a).
[734] Swart and Keulartz (2011).
[735] See Mellor (2015).
[736] Dawkins (1990).

disturbance as a result of human interference. Land clearing, for pasture creation, mining, forestry and so on, is particularly deleterious to the welfare of wild animals. Animals may be killed or injured during the clearing itself, they may suffer when debris is burned, and longer term they may have difficulty surviving in the changed or lost habitat. It has been estimated that about 50 million mammals, birds and reptiles are killed each year as a result of land clearing in New South Wales and Queensland.[737] There is now scientific consensus that habitat loss resulting from land clearing is the number one threat to Australia's native species.[738]

Meddling with wildlife is not just at the level of that interaction with habitat. Conservation has become popular; this has manifest itself with studies of wild animals, which studies can themselves be invasive and have negative impacts on their subjects, as well as more aggressive interventions to preserve species under threat. In this latter case, those interventions can involve the destruction of other native (and feral) animals. Wild animals have been introduced or re-introduced in an effort to restore damaged natural areas. This is not necessarily a good thing for the introduced animals.[739] There is no doubt that by using and contaminating land and water, agriculture is a greater threat to wildlife and biodiversity than any other human activity.[740]

Wildlife comes a poor second to human commercial interests, particularly those concerned with farming. During the expansion of settlement in Australia, it is evident that there was wholesale slaughter of native animals to prevent them feeding on the immigrants' crops.[741] It has been said that large predators are declining as a result of hunting and killing activities driven by the livestock industry. It is an article of

---

[737] Finn and Stephens (2017).
[738] Wintle and Bekessy. 'Let's get this straight, habitat loss is the number-one threat to Australia's species'. *The Conversation* 17 October 2017.
[739] Swart and Keulartz (2011).
[740] Garnett et al. (2013).
[741] Franklin (2007a).

faith for farmers that farm animals need to be protected from predators, so predators have to be killed.

The dingo is an animal which has gone from being despised and pursued, to being the subject of reclassification by the 'eco-nationalism' tendency. It is now regarded as a native animal – in other words it was here before Western settlement of Australia in 1788. But this rehabilitation has been short-lived. Dingoes (like many wild animals) can be dangerous, and when they attack people, the tendency is to declare them to be pests.[742] Indeed, in Australia, many jurisdictions have declared dingoes to be pests. In Queensland, for example, 'wild dogs' are defined under the *Biosecurity Act 2014* to include dingoes. The upshot of that is that dingoes can be trapped, poisoned (1080 - sodium fluoroactetate, strychnine, para amino propiophenone) or shot. Several councils in Queensland offer bounties for dingoes. There is a similar situation in New South Wales, where dingoes are declared pests under the *Local Land Services Act 2013*. This places an obligation on the managers of rural land to eradicate them. Note, however, that in an act of schizophrenia, dingoes qualify for consideration as threatened species under the New South Wales *Threatened Species Conservation Act 1995*, as they were established in the state before European settlement. Contrary to simplistic analyses, there is evidence to suggest that where dingoes are left to their own devices, the leading causes of death of cattle in remote rangeland farms in central Australia were 'husbandry-related challenges' and deteriorating environmental conditions. Predation by dingoes was a minor cause. In any case, there is evidence that attempts at lethal control of dingoes can cause increases in both dingo population density (by loss of reproductive suppression) and predation rates.[743]

A footnote to this is that wildlife ecologists take the view that, as the largest mammalian predator in the country, dingoes limit the densities

---

[742] Franklin (2007a).
[743] Wallach et al. (2017).

of wild herbivores, such as kangaroos and goats. They are also known to reduce populations of foxes and cats. This again illustrates the confused attitude of those obsessed with eradication of 'pests'. Sometimes the pests you eradicate are controlling populations of other pests, so in eradicating the first pest, you increase the population of the second pest.

Kangaroos are killed in Australia for commercial gain, as well as for fun and to stop them eating farmers' grass.[744] Most kangaroos shot are males, but when females are shot they will usually have either or both pouch young or young at foot. Something like 20-30% of kangaroos shot are females and perhaps one fifth of those have young at foot. This may represent perhaps 600,000 animals in the period from 1999 to 2012. Interestingly, there has been a drop in female kangaroos killed in 2012, ostensibly due to one kangaroo processor accepting only male carcases, in response to public concern about the welfare of orphaned joeys. But this seems to have been associated with almost doubling of the number of female kangaroos killed by non-commercial shooters. Sharp and MacLeod (2016) reported a very limited survey of commercial kangaroo killers in New South Wales. Despite its limitations, this survey found from those kangaroo killers who were observed (as opposed to asked questions) that there was very little done in the way of complying with the relevant Code and killing young at foot after the mother had been killed. Astonishing to think that shooters under observation just disobeyed the law. Imagine what they do when they are not being watched.

It is a statement of the obvious to say that the most humane way to kill a kangaroo is to shoot it in the head. Given the vagaries of shooting wild animals at night (when the shooting is done), it is equally obvious that this may not be what happens in the real world. What is needed, and

---

[744] see Chapter 10; Descovich et al. (2015).

what has never been done, are field-based surveys to find out what actually does happen.[745]

It appears that Tasmania is the only Australian jurisdiction where it is lawful to poison macropods (ie wallabies) with 1080.

---

[745] Descovich et al. (2015).

# Chapter 14  The way forward

It is easy to become despondent about the swings back and forth regarding animal welfare in Australia. At the moment we are firmly in the 'backlash' phase, where the farming lobby and others who make money out of animal use are getting their way more and more. I am heartened, however, by the words of John Webster, who has been involved in this area longer and at a greater depth than I:

> '...it is better to limp towards Eden step by step than to retire to the comfort of the moral high ground and cry havoc on all who live in the real world.'[746]

Having said that, however, I think what we must emphasise in Australia is there will only be improvement if those with vested interests are excluded from the advice-giving process so far as animal welfare policy is concerned. That is not to say that commercial interests should have no say, but they should not be involved at the initial stages. Setting out the way forward for animal welfare can initially be defined by science, then modified by economic reality and ethical considerations, and ultimately decided on, taking all these things into account. by the people whose job it is – the politicians.

The disproportionate influence of the animal use industry in setting and administering policy is seen in the nature of government departments involved in making and enforcing laws dealing with animals. Federally, the most important laws concerning animal welfare are those relating to live export and killing of animals to provide products (principally meat) for export. That is dealt with by the Department of Agriculture and Water Resources. The States and Territories Departments which are responsible have as their main aim the promotion of agriculture, that is, animal exploitation.

The conclusion is that every government department which should be concerned with looking after the welfare of animals is hopelessly

---

[746] Webster (2005).

compromised and conflicted by their primary role, which is to look after the interests of those who make money out of animals. This was expressly noted by (then) federal Labor MP Melissa Parke at the National Conference in 2011.[747]

In 2008 I wrote 'what is needed is a completely independent, nationally-based animal welfare commission, with responsibility for advising on legislation and enforcement.'[748] This has since been echoed by many.[749]

I suggested this required concerted effort and cooperation between the federal and states governments. Federal Agriculture Minister Barnaby Joyce has set things back considerably in this regard by removing the federal government from any general role in animal welfare. The current two party system is unlikely to see any significant change in the foreseeable future, as both parties appear incapable of doing anything which they think will upset farmers. This amounts to animal welfare paralysis.

Astonishingly, the Productivity Commission (an independent government agency which advises on economic matters) has released a report proposing the establishment of 'an independent statutory agency – the Australian Commission for Animal Welfare – to develop the national standards and guidelines'. This Commission would disseminate information on best practice farm animal husbandry, including through further development of the standards and guidelines.[750] The proposed Commission should also regularly review the performance of the ESCAS system in the live export trade.

It is more than obvious that the decisions relating to animal welfare must be made by politicians, and those politicians need to be informed by independently-assessed animal welfare science. By that I mean

---

[747] Cited in Goodfellow (2015).
[748] Caulfield (2008).
[749] See Goodfellow (2015).
[750] Productivity Commission (2017) *Regulation of Australian Agriculture*. Report No 79.

where particular issues are under consideration, such as (for example) keeping chickens in battery cages, the first step should be a review of the relevant animal welfare science by scientists who are truly independent of industry. What this means in practical terms is that those scientists who have built their careers on industry-funded research will have difficulty proving their independence. Unfortunately, in Australia, much of the animal welfare science research referring to matters concerning farm animals is paid for by industry, so scientists wishing to advance their career are forced to take the industry shilling.

The issue of independent scientific advice is not as thorny as it may appear. There is a wealth of information available from international sources, most of it relevant to the Australian scene. The most obvious example is the animal welfare function of the European Food Safety Authority, which publishes well-researched and reliable information on many important animal welfare issues. This should be the first port of call in assessing any animal welfare situation under consideration for regulation. As unbelievable as it may seem, for many years leading Australian animal welfare scientists have persisted in claiming that so far as farm animals are concerned, there is a need for 'Australian animal welfare science' to be done before any decisions can be made regarding changes. Unless the particular Australian system is unique (and live export is one such example), then science from the rest of the world is almost inevitably going to be relevant. To pretend otherwise is sophistry.

This may all be pie in the sky, because what is clear is that the average Australian wants improvements in animal welfare, but their elected representatives (that is, those in the Liberal – National coalition and the Labor Party) are not prepared to give it to them. This is a defect of our version of democracy. Because good animal welfare, even though valued, is too low down the list of voter priorities, it doesn't get a mention. The politicians, however, are becoming less and less in favour. People are completely disenchanted with the say everything, do nothing flavour of modern politics. The religiously-oriented right wing has profited by this and it is surely only a matter of time before those who are of a more compassionate nature will use public disenchantment to demand their share of the newly sliced-up political pie. This may be in the form of an increased vote for the Greens (but I doubt it), or it may be in the form of one-issue parties securing a position from which they can exert political leverage. I am not holding my breath, but things do seem to be heading in the direction of less political stability, which can only mean potential for change. Who then, is going to push the change?

In the last couple of years I have been privileged to work closely with young lawyers who have set up the Animal Law Institute. I am their Principal Solicitor. This organisation is able to offer free legal advice (and indeed run law cases) for those pursuing animal welfare issues. These are highly professional, educated, enthusiastic people; unsurprisingly, they are mostly women. This is the future. The educated youth of today are less and less likely, in my view, to make the mistakes their forebears made regarding animal welfare. The increasing involvement of women in positions of power and influence will, I believe, result in a steady improvement.

# Bibliography

ABARES [Australian Bureau of Agricultural and Resource Economics and Sciences] (2016) *Agricultural commodity statistics 2016*.

Abbey, R (2007) Rawlsian resources for animal ethics. *Ethics & the Environment* 12:1-22.

ABS [Australian Bureau of Statistics] (2015) *National Health Survey* (cat no 4364.0.55.001).

ABS [Australian Bureau of Statistics] (2016) *Australian Health Survey: consumption of food groups from the Australian Dietary Guidelines* (cat no 4364.0.55.012).

Acampora, R. (2016) Provocations from the field – Epistemology of ignorance and human privilege. *Animal Studies Journal* 5:1-20.

Adams, CJ (2010) *The sexual politics of meat: a feminist-vegetarian critical theory*. Bloomsbury (20th anniversary edition).

ACIL Tasman (2009) *The value of live sheep exports from Western Australia*.

Albright, KM (2002) The extension of legal rights to animals under a caring ethic: an ecofeminist exploration of Steven Wise's *Rattling the Cage*. *Natural Resources Journal* 42:916-937.

Algers B et al. (2005). Opinion of the Scientific Panel on Animal Health and Welfare on a request from the Commission related to the welfare aspects of various systems of keeping laying hens. *EFSA J* 197:1-23.

Algers, B et al. (2007) Animal health and welfare aspects of different housing and husbandry systems for adult breeding boars, pregnant, farrowing sows and unweaned piglets. *EFSA Journal* 572:1-3.

Anderson, EC and Feldman Barrett, L (2016) Affective beliefs influence the experience of eating meat. *PLOS One* 11 e0160424; doi:10.1371/journal.pone.0160424.

Anil, L et al. (2002) Relationship between postural behaviour and gestation stall dimensions in relation to sow size *Applied Animal Behaviour Science* 77:173-181.

Arkow, P (2012) Foreword to Gullone (2012).

Arlinghaus, R et al. (2012) A primer on anti-angling philosophy and its relevance for recreational fisheries in urbanized societies. *Fisheries* 37:153-164.

Australian Egg Corporation Limited (2016) *Australian egg industry overview – December 2015*.

Baars, BJ and Edelman, DB (2012) Consciousness, biology and quantum hypotheses. *Physics of Life Reviews* 9:285-294.

Bargheer, S (2006) The fools of the leisure class. Honor, ridicule, and the emergence of animal protection legislation in England, 1740-1840. *European Journal of Sociology* 47:3-35.

Barrett, J et al. (2014) Smothering in UK free-range flocks. Part 1: incidence, location, timing and management. *Veterinary Record* doi:10.1136/vr.102327.

Barnett, JL and Hemsworth, PH (1990) The validity of physiological and behavioural measures of animal welfare. *Applied Animal Behaviour Science* 25:177-187.

Barnett, JL et al. (2001) A review of the welfare issues for sows and piglets in relation to housing. *Australian Journal of Agricultural Research* 52:1-28.

Barton MD (2000) Antibiotic use in animal feed and its impact on human health. *Nutrition Research Reviews* 13:279-299.

Bastian, B. et al. (2012) Don't mind meat? The denial of mind to animals used for human consumption. *Personality and Social Psychology Bulletin* 38: 247-256.

Benson, GJ and Rollin, BE (2004) *The well-being of farm animals – challenges and solutions*. Blackwell Publishing.

Beausoleil J et al. (2016) A systematic approach to evaluating and ranking the relative animal welfare impacts of wildlife control methods: poisons used for lethal control of brushtail possums (*Trichosurus vulpecula*) in New Zealand. *Wildlife Research* 43:553-565.

Bergstrom, DM et al. (2009) Indirect effects of invasive species removal devastate World Heritage Island. *Journal of Applied Ecology* 46:73-81.

Blokhuis, HJ (2008) International cooperation in animal welfare: the Welfare Quality project. *Acta Veterinaria Scandinavica* 50:S10.

Botterill, LC (2007) Managing intergovernmental relations in Australia: the case of agricultural policy cooperation. *The Australian Journal of Public Administration* 66:186-197.

Bouvard, V et al. (2015) Carcinogenicity of consumption of red and processed meat. *Lancet Oncology* 16:1599-1600.

Bowen, A and Casadevall, A (2015) Increasing disparities between resource inputs and outcomes, as measured by certain health deliverables, in biomedical research. *Proceedings of the National Academy of Sciences* 112:11335-11340.

Bloom, G (2008) Regulating animal welfare to promote and protect improved animal welfare outcomes under the Australian Animal Welfare Strategy. Commissioned by the Department of Agriculture.

Bonnie, KE et al. (2016) Effects of crowd size on exhibit use by and behavior of chimpanzees (*Pan troglodytes*) and Western lowland gorillas (*Gorilla gorilla*) at a zoo. *Applied Animal Behaviour Science* 178:102-110.

Boutron, I et al. (2010) Reporting and interpretation of randomized controlled trials with statistically nonsignificant results for primary outcomes. *JAMA* 303:2058-2064.

Bray, HJ and Ankeny, RA (2017) Happy chickens lay tastier eggs: motivations for buying free-range eggs in Australia. *Anthrozoos* 30:213-226.

Brody, T (1999) *Nutritional Biochemistry*. Academic Press.

Broom, DM (1986) Indicators of poor welfare. *British Veterinary Journal* 142: 624-526.

Broom, DM (1996) Animal welfare defined in terms of attempts to cope with the environment. *Acta Agriculturae Scandinavica Section A, Animal Science: Supplement* 27:22-28.

Broom, DM (2003) *The evolution of morality and religion*. Cambridge University Press.

Broom, DM (2006) The evolution of morality. *Applied Animal Behaviour Science* 100:20-28.

Broom (2007) Cognitive ability and sentience: which aquatic animals should be protected? *Diseases of Aquatic Organisms* 75:99-108.

Broom, DM (2009) Animal welfare and legislation. in *Welfare of production animals: assessment and management of risks*. Academic Publishers.

Broom, DM (2011) A history of animal welfare science. *Acta Biotheoretica* 59:121-137.

Broom, DM (2014) *Sentience and animal welfare*. CABI.

Broom, DM and Fraser, AG. (2007) *Domestic animal behaviour and welfare*. (4th edition). CABI.

Bruce, A (2012) *Animal law in Australia: an integrated approach*. LexisNexis Butterworths.

Burghardt, GM (2007) Critical anthropomorphism, uncritical anthropomorphism and naive nominalism. *Comparative Cognition & Behavior Reviews* 2:136-138.

Burghardt, GM (2016) Mediating claims through critical anthropomorphism. *Animal Sentience* 2016.024.

Campbell, DLM et al. (2016) fear and coping styles of outdoor-preferring, moderate-outdoor and indoor-preferring free-range laying hens. *Applied Animal Behaviour Science* 185:73-77.

Caple I et al. (2010). *Live Trade Animal Welfare Partnership 2009/10; Indonesian point of slaughter improvements*. MLA / LiveCorp.

Casal, P (2003) Is multiculturalism bad for animals? *The Journal of Political Philosophy* 11:1-22.

Caulfield, M (2008) *Animal cruelty law in Australia*. Animals Australia.

Caulfield, M (2013) *Science and sense – the case for abolishing sow stalls*. Voiceless.

Caulfield, M (2017) How the Australian animal use industry employs arguments against anthropomorphism, coupled with bad science, to skew animal welfare law. *Animal Studies Journal* 6:155-174.

Caulfield, MP and Cambridge, H (2008) The questionable value of some science-based 'welfare' assessments in intensive animal farming: sow stalls as an illustrative example. *Australian Veterinary Journal* 86:446-448.

Caulfield, MP et al. (2014) Heat stress: a major contributor to poor animal welfare associated with long-haul live export voyages. *The Veterinary Journal* 199:223-228.

Chen, PJ (2016) *Animal welfare in Australia*. Sydney University Press.

Collignon P (2004) Antibiotic growth promoters *Journal of Antimicrobial Chemotherapy* DOI:10.1093/jac/dkh266

Collignon P (2012) Does antibiotic use in farmed animals pose a risk to human health? *Medical Journal of Australia* 196:302.

Collignon P (2015) Antibiotic resistance: are we all doomed? *Internal Medicine Journal* 45:1109-1115.

Colquhoun, D (1971) *Lectures on Biostatistics*. Clarendon Press.

Colquhoun, D (2014) An investigation of the false discovery rate and the misinterpretation of *p*-values. *Royal Society Open Science* 1:140216 www.dx.doi.org/10.1098/rsos.140216.

Comrie, N (2016) *Independent review of the RSPCA Victoria Inspectorate* www.rspcavic.org/documents/RSPCA_IndependentReview_final.pdf.

Cooke, SJ and Sneddon LU (2006) Animal wefare perspective on recreational angling. *Applied Animal Behaviour Science* 104:176-198.

Cornish, P et al. (2016) What we know about the public's level of concern for farm animal welfare in food production in developed countries. *Animals* 6:74.

Dalziell, J and Wadiwei, DJ (2017) Live exports, animal advocacy, race and 'animal nationalism'. In *Meat Culture*. ed A Potts; Brill.

Darwin, C (1871) *The descent of man and selection in relation to sex* see https://en.wikisource.org/wiki/The_Descent_of_Man_(Darwin).

Davis, K (2017) The provocative elitism of 'personhood' for nonhuman creatures in animal advocacy parlance and polemics. In *Meat Culture*. ed. A Potts; Brill.

Dawkins, MS (1990) From an animal's point of view: motivation, fitness and animal welfare. *Behavioral and Brain Sciences* 13:1-8.

Dawkins, MS (2006) Through animal eyes: what behaviour tells us. *Applied Animal Behaviour Science* 100:4-10.

Dawkins, MS (2017a) Animal welfare with and without consciousness *Journal of Zoology* 301:1-10.

Dawkins, MS (2017b) Animal welfare and efficient farming: is conflict inevitable? *Animal Production Science* 57:201-208.

D'Eath, RB and Turner, SP (2009) The natural behaviour of the pig, in *The Welfare of Pigs*. Springer Science + Business Direct.

Degeling, C and Johnson, J (2015) Citizens, consumers and animals: what role do experts assign to public values in establishing animal welfare standards? *Journal of Agricultural and Environmental Ethics* 28:961-976.

Descovich, KA et al. (2015) A welfare assessment of methods used for harvesting, hunting and population control of kangaroos and wallabies. *Animal Welfare* 24:255-265.

de Waal, FBM (2008) Putting the altruism back into altruism: the evolution of empathy. *Annual Review of Psychology* 59:279-300.

Dhont, K et al. (2016) Common ideological roots of speciesism and generalized ethnic prejudice: the social dominance human-animal relations model (SD-HARM). *European Journal of Personality* 30:507-522.

Diggles, BK (2016) Development of resources to promote best practice in the humane dispatch of finfish caught by recreational fishers. Fisheries Management and Ecology 23:200-207.

Dilworth, T and McGregor, A (2015) Moral steaks? Ethical discourses of in vitro meat in academia and Australia. *Journal of Agricultural and Environmental Ethics* 28:85-107.

Doherty, TS et al. (2015a) Multiple threats, or multiplying the threats? Interactions between invasive predators and other ecological disturbances. *Biological Conservation* 190:60-68.

Doherty, TS et al. (2015b) A continental-scale analysis of feral cat diet in Australia. *Journal of Biogeography* 42:964-975.

Doherty, TS et al. (2016) Impacts and management of feral cats *Felis catus* in Australia. *Mammal Review* 47:83-97.

Doherty, TS and Ritchie, EG (2017) Stop jumping the gun: a call for evidence-based invasive predator management. *Conservation Letters* 10:16-22.

Dorning, J et al (2016) *The welfare of wild animals in travelling circuses*. www.ispca.ie/uploads/The_welfare_of_wild_animals_in_travelling_circus es.pdf

Dowling, CE et al. (2010) Immediate fate of angled-and-released Australian bass *Macquaria novemaculeata*. *Hydrobiologia* 641:145-157.

Duncan, IJH (2006) The changing concept of sentience. *Applied Animal Behaviour Science* 100:11-19.

Duncan, IJH and Petherick, JC (1991) The implications of cognitive processes for animal welfare. *Journal of Animal Science* 69:5017-5022.

Durham, TB and Blanco, M-J (2015) Target engagement in lead generation. *Bioorganic and Medicinal Chemistry Letters* 25:998-1008.

Eason, CT et al. (2010) Advancing a humane alternative to sodium fluoroacetate (1080) for wildlife management – welfare and wallaby control. *Wildlife Research* 37:497-503.

Edelman, DB and Seth, AK (2009) Animal consciousness: a synthetic approach. *Trends in Neurosciences* 32:476-484.

Ellis, E (2012) Bearing the burden: shifting responsibility for the welfare of the beast. *Macquarie Law Journal* 11:39-49.

Elson, HA (2015) Poultry welfare in intensive and extensive production systems. *World's Poultry Science Journal* 71:449-460.

Enna, SJ and Williams, M (2009) Challenges in the search for drugs to treat central nervous system disorders. *Journal of Pharmacology and Experimental Therapeutics* 329:404-411.

Eshel, G (2014) Land, irrigation water, greenhouse gas, and reactive nitrogen burdens of meat, eggs, and dairy production in the United States. *Proceedings of the National Academy of Sciences (USA)* 111:11996-12001.

Fancourt, BA and Jackson, RB (2014) Regional seroprevalence of *Toxoplasma gondii* antibodies in feral and stray cats (*Felis catus*) from Tasmania. *Australian Journal of Zoology* 62:272-283.

FAO [Food and Agriculture Organisation of the United Nations] (2006) *Livestock's Long Shadow*.

Ferter, K et al. (2017) Survival of Atlantic halibut (*Hippoglossus hippoglossus*) following catch-and-release angling. *Fisheries Research* 186:634-641.

Finch, N et al. (2014) Expenditure and motivation of Australian recreational hunters. *Wildlife Research* 41:76-83.

Finn, HC and Stephens, NS (2017) The invisible harm: land clearing is an issue of animal welfare. *Wildlife Research* doi:10.1071/WR17018.

Fisher et al. (2014) The effects of direct and indirect road transport consignment in combination with feed withdrawal in young dairy calves. *Journal of Dairy Research* 81:297-303.

Fitzgerald, AJ et al (2009) Slaughterhouses and increased crime rates. An empirical analysis of the spillover from 'the jungle' into the surrounding community. *Organization & Environment* 22:158-184.

Francione, GL (1995) *Animals, property and the law*. Temple University Press.

Francione, GL (2000 *Introduction to animal rights*. Temple University Press.

Franklin, A (2007a) *Animal Nation*. UNSW Press.

Franklin, A (2007b) Human-nonhuman animal relationships in Australia: an overview of results from the first national survey and follow-up case studies 2000-2004. *Society and Animals* 15:7-27.

Franklin, RG et al (2013) Neural responses to perceiving suffering in humans and animals. *Social Neuroscience* 8:217-227.

Fraser, D (2012) A 'practical' ethic for animals. *Journal of Agricultural and Environmental Ethics* 25:721-746.

Fraser, D et al. (2013) General principles for the welfare of animals in production systems: the underlying science and its application. *The Veterinary Journal* 198:19-27.

Freire, R and Cowling, A (2013) The welfare of laying hens in conventional cages and alternative systems: first steps towards a quantitative comparison. *Animal Welfare* 22: 57-65.

Fuseini A et al (2016) The stunning and slaughter of cattle within the EU: a review of the current situation with regard to the halal market. *Animal Welfare* 25:365-376.

Gale, CR (2006) IQ in childhood and vegetarianism in adulthood: 1970 British cohort study. *British Medical Journal* doi:10.1136/bmj.39030.675069.55.

Garner, R (2002) Political ideology and the legal status of animals. *Animal Law* 8:77-91.

Garnett, T et al. (2013) Sustainable intensification in agriculture: premises and policies. *Science* 341:33-34.

Garrett, A (2007) Francis Hutcheson and the origin of animal rights. *Journal of the History of Philosophy* 45:243-265.

Gershell, LJ and Atkins, JH (2003) A brief history of novel drug discovery technologies. *Nature Reviews Drug Discovery* 2:321-327.

Goncalves, J et al. (2014) The risks of using 'species-specific' PCR assays in wildlife research: the case of red fox (*Vulpes vulpes*) identification in Tasmania. *Forensic Science International: Genetics* 11:e9-e11.

Goodfellow, J (2015) *Animal welfare regulation in the Australian agricultural sector: a legitimacy maximising analysis*. PhD thesis, Macquarie University.

Grandin T (1997) Assessment of stress during handling and transport. *Journal of Animal Science* 75:249.

Grandin T (2010) *Recommended animal handling guidelines and audit guide: a systematic approach to animal welfare*. American Meat Institute Foundation.

Grandin T (2013) Making slaughterhouses more humane for cattle, pigs and sheep. *Annual Review of Animal Bioscience* 1:491-512.

Green, TC and Mellor, DJ (2011) Extending ideas about animal welfare assessment to include 'quality of life' and related concepts. *New Zealand Veterinary Journal* 59:316-324.

Grethe, H (2007) High animal welfare standards in the EU and international trade – how to prevent potential 'low animal welfare havens'? *Food Policy* 32:315-333.

Griffin, E (2007) *Blood Sport – Hunting in Britain since 1066*. Yale University Press.

Gross, D and Tolba, RH (2015) Ethics in animal-based research. *European Surgical Research* 55:43-57.

Guesgen, MJ et al. (2011) The effects of age and sex on pain sensitivity in young lambs. *Applied Animal Behaviour Science* 135:51-56.

Gullone, E. (2012) *Animal cruelty, antisocial behaviour and aggression*. Palgrave Macmillan.

Gullone, E (2015) Recreational hunting, animal cruelty, aggression against humans: what's the difference? https//eleonoragullone.wordpress.com/2015/01/09/recreational-hunting-animal-cruelty-aggression-against-humans-whats-the-difference/.

Hackam, DG and Redelmeier, DA (2006) Translation of research evidence from animals to humans. *Journal of the American Medical Association* 296:1727-1732.

Hagan, K et al. (2011) Concepts of animal welfare. *Acta Biotheoretica* 59:93-109.

Hall, CM et al. (2016) Do collar-mounted predation deterrents restrict wandering in pet domestic cats? *Applied Animal Behaviour Science* 176:96-104.

Harrison, R (1964) *Animal machines: the new factory farming*. Vincent Stuart.

Haynes, R (2011) Competing conceptions of animal welfare and their ethical implications for the treatment of non-human animals. *Acta Biotheoretica* 59:105-120.

Heaney, RP et al. (2000) Bioavailability of the calcium in fortified soy imitation milk, with some observations on method. *American Journal of Clinical Nutrition* 71:1166-1169.

Held, S et al. (2009) Advances in the study of cognition, behavioural priorities and emotions, in *The Welfare of Pigs*. Springer Science + Business Direct.

Hemmila, IA and Hurskainen, P (2002) Novel detection strategies for drug discovery. *DDT* 7:S150-S156.

Hemsworth, PH et al. (2013) Effects of group size and floor space allowance on grouped sows: aggression, stress, skin injuries and reproductive performance. *Journal of Animal Science* 91:4953-4964.

Hemsworth, PH et al. (2015) Scientific assessment of animal welfare. *New Zealand Veterinary Journal* 63:24-30.

Herwig, A (2016) Too much zeal on seals' animal welfare, public morals and consumer ethics at the bar of the WTO. *World Trade Review* 15:109-137.

Herzog, HA (2007) Gender differences in human-animal interactions: a review. *Anthrozoos* 20:7-21.

Heuer OE et al. (2009) Human health consequences of use of antimicrobial agents in aquaculture. *Clinical Infectious Diseases* 49:1248-53.

Holdier, AG (2016) The pig's squeak: towards a renewed aesthetic agrument for veganism. *Journal of Agricultural and Environmental Ethics* 29:631-642.

Hood, J et al. (2017) Whip rule breaches in a major Australian racing jurisdiction: welfare and regulatory implications. *Animals* 7:4.

Hoogland, CT et al. (2005) Transparency of the meat chain in the light of food culture and history. *Appetite* 45:15-23.

Horrobin, DF (2003) Modern biomedical research: an internally self-consistent universe with little contact with medical reality? *Nature Reviews Drug Discovery* 2:151-154.

Hughes, PE et al. (2010) Relationships among gilt and sow live weight, P2 backfat depth, and culling rates. *Journal of Swine Health Production* 84:1004-1014.

Humane Research Council [now known as 'Faunalytics'] (2014) *Animal Tracker Australia*.

Ioannidis, JPA (2005) Why most published research findings are false. *PLoS Medicine* 2:696-701.

Jarvis, MF and Williams, M (2016) Irreproducibility in preclinical biomedical research; perceptions, uncertainties and knowledge gaps. *Trends in Pharmacological Sciences* 37:290-302.

Jechalke S et al. (2014) Fate and effects of veterinary antibiotics in the soil. *Trends in Microbiology* 22:536-545

Jones, B and Davies, J. (2016) *Backlash*. Finlay Lloyd Publishers.

Jordan D et al. (2009) Antimicrobial use in the Australian pig industry: results of a national survey. *Australian Veterinary Journal* 87:222-229.

Joy, M. (2010) *Why we love dogs, eat pigs and wear cows*. Conari Press.

Kannt, A and Wieland, T (2016) Managing risks in drug discovery: reproducibility of published findings. *Naunyn-Schmiedebergs Archives of Pharmacology* 389:353-360.

Kean, H (1998) *Animal rights*. Reaktion Books.

Kelch, TG (2016) Towards universal principles for global animal advocacy. *Transnational Environmental Law* 5:81-111.

Kenakin, R (2013) Replicated, replicable and relevant – target engagement and pharmacological experimentation in the 21st century. *Biochemical Pharmacology* 87:64-77.

Kennedy, JS (1992) *The new anthropomorphism*. Cambridge University Press.

Kheel, M (1996) The killing game: an ecofeminist critique of hunting. *Journal of the Philosophy of Sport* 23:30-44.

Kildal, CL and Syse, KL (2017) Meat and masculinity in the Norwegian armed forces. *Appetite*112:69-77.

Kiley-Worthington, M (2016) Book review: The welfare of performing animals. A historical perspective. *Animals* 6:76; doi:10.3390/ani6110076.

Kirkwood, J (2006) The distribution of the capacity for sentience in the animal kingdom. in *Animals, ethics and trade; the challenge of animal sentience*. eds J Turner and J D'Silva, Compassion in World Farming Trust.

Kohlenberg-Mueller, K and Raschka, L (2003) Calcium balance in young adults on a vegan and lactovegetarian diet. *Journal of Bone and Mineral Metabolism* 21:28-33.

Kupsala, S et al. (2013) Who cares about farmed fish? Citizen perceptions of the welfare and the mental abilities of fish. *Journal of Agricultural and Environmental Ethics*. 26:119-135.

Larsen, H et al. (2017) Individual ranging behaviour patterns in commercial free-range layers as observed through RFID tracking. *Animals* 7,21 doi:10.3390/ani/7030021.

Laurikssens, B (2013) Animal models of Alzheimer's disease and drug development. *Drug Discovery Today: Technologies* 10:e319-e327.

Lay DC et al. (2011) Hen welfare in different housing systems. *Poultry Science* 90:278-294.

Lay, DC and Marchant-Forde, JN (2009) Future perspectives of the welfare of pigs, in *The Welfare of Pigs*. Springer Science + Business Direct.

Layton-Bennett, A (2014) 3000 sightings later, Tasmania seeks fox proof. *The Veterinarian* May 2014, 3.

Lazebnik, Y (2015) Are scientists a workforce? – Or, how Dr Frankenstein made biomedical research sick. *EMBO Reports* 16:1592-1600.

Lazenby, BT et al. (2015) Effects of low-level culling of feral cats in open populations: a case study from the forests of southern Tasmania. *Wildlife Research* 41:407-420.

Legge, S et al. (2017) Enumerating a continental-scale threat: how many feral cats are in Australia? *Biological Conservation* 206:293-303.

Littin, K et al. (2014) Welfare aspects of vertebrate pest control and culling: ranking control techniques for humaneness. *Revue Scientifique et Technique* 33:281-289.

Littin, KE et al. (2004) Animal welfare and ethical issues relevant to the humane control of vertebrate pests. *New Zealand Veterinary Journal* 52:1-10.

Littin, KE et al. (2009) Behaviour and time to unconsciousness of brushtail possums (*Trichosurus vulpecula*) after a lethal or sublethal dose of 1080. *Wildlife Research* 36:709-720.

Lomax, S. et al. (2013) Duration of action of a topical anaesthetic formulation for pain management of mulesing in sheep. *Australian Veterinary Journal* 91:160-167.

Lovvorn, JR (2006) Animal law in action: the law, public perception and the limits of animal rights theory as a basis for legal reform. *Animal Law* 12:133-149.

Lund, TB et al. (2016) Animal ethics profiling of vegetarians, vegans and meat-eaters. *Anthrozoos* 29:89-106.

McBride, G et al. (1969) The social organization and behaviour of the feral domestic fowl. *Animal Behaviour Monographs* 2:125-180.

McGlone, JJ et al. (2004) The physical size of gestating sows *Journal of Animal Science* 82:2421-2427.

McGreevy, PD et al (2012) Whip use by jockeys in a sample of Australian thoroughbred races – an observational study. *Plos One* 7:e33398; doi:10.1371/journal.pone.0033398

McHugh, M. (2016) *Special Commission of Inquiry into the Greyhound Racing Industry in NSW.* www.greyhoundracinginquiry.justice.nsw.gov.au

McLean, AN and McGreevy, PD (2010) Ethical equitation: capping the price horses pay for human glory. *Journal of Veterinary Behavior* 5:203-209.

Mathijs, E (2015) Exploring future patterns of meat consumption. *Meat Science* 109:112-116.

Maloni, MJ and Brown, ME (2006) Corporate social responsibility in the supply chain: an application in the food industry. *Journal of Business Ethics* 68:35-52.

Marchant-Forde, JN (2009a) Introduction, in *The Welfare of Pigs*. Springer Science + Business Direct.

Marchant-Forde, JN (2009b) Welfare of dry sows, in *The Welfare of Pigs*. Springer Science + Business Direct.

Marino, L (2016) Thinking chickens: a review of cognition, emotion, and behaviour in the domestic chicken. *Animal Cognition* 20:127-147.

Melina, V et al. (2015) Position of the Academy of Nutrition and Dietetics: vegetarian diets. *Journal of the Academy of Nutrition and Dietetics* 116:1870-1980.

Mellor, DJ (2015) Positive animal welfare states and reference standards for welfare assessment. *New Zealand Veterinary Journal* 63:17-23.

Mellor, DJ and Beausoleil, NJ (2015) Extending the 'Five Domains' model for animal welfare assessment to incorporate positive welfare states. *Animal Welfare* 24:241-253.

Mellor, DJ (2016a) Moving beyond the 'Five Freedoms' by updating the 'Five Provisions' and introducing aligned 'Animal Welfare Aims'. *Animals* 6,1-7.

Mellor, DJ (2016b) Updating animal welfare thinking: moving beyond the 'five freedoms' towards a 'life worth living'. *Animals* 6:21.

Mill, JS (1843) *System of logic, deductive and inductive*. Longman.

Mormede, P et al. (2007) Exploration of the hypothalamic-pituitary-adrenal function as a tool to evaluate animal welfare. *Physiology & Behaviour* 92:317-339.

Morisse, JP et al. (1995) Effect of dehorning on behaviour and plasma cortisol responses in young calves. *Applied Animal Behaviour Science* 43:229-247.

Motulsky, HJ (2015) Common misconceptions about data analysis and statistics. *British Journal of Pharmacology* 172:2126-2132.

Mullane, K and Williams, M (2015) Unknown unknowns in biomedical research: does an inability to deal with ambiguity contribute to issues of irreproducibility? *Biochemical Pharmacology* 97:133-136.

Mullee, A et al. (2017) Vegetarianism and meat consumption: a comparison of attitudes and beliefs between vegetarian, semi-vegetarian and omnivorous subjects in Belgium. *Appetite* 114:299-305.

NHMRC (National Health and Medical Research Council) (2013) *Australian Dietary Guidelines*.

Nicol, CJ et al. (2017) *Farmed Bird Welfare Science Review* published by the Department of Economic Development, Jobs, Transport and Resources, Victoria.

Neumann, G and Associates (2005) Review of the Australian Model Codes of Practice for the Welfare of Animals.

Norman, GJ (2016) *National livestock export industry sheep, cattle and goat transport performance report 2015*. Meat and Livestock Australia report W.LIV.0291.

Nussbaum, M (2006) *Frontiers of justice. Disability, nationality, species membership*. Belknap Press of the Harvard University Press.

O'Connell, MK et al. (2007) Measuring changes in physical size and predicting weight of sows during gestation. *Animal* 1:1335-1343.

O'Sullivan, S (2012) *Animals, equality and democracy*. Palgrave.

Pardes, H et al. (1991) Physicians and the animal-rights movement. *The New England Journal of Medicine* 324:1640-1643.

Parbery, P and Wilkinson, R *Victorians' attitudes to farming*. Department of Primary Industries.

Paull, DR et al. (2007) The effect of a topical anaesthetic formulation, systemic flunixin and carprofen, singly or in combination, on cortisol and behavioural responses of Merino lambs to mulesing. *Australian Veterinary Journal* 85: 98-106.

Pearson, A et al. (2007) Animals and the law in Australia: a livestock industry perspective. *Reform* 91:25-29.

Pendergrast, N. (2015) Live animal export, humane slaughter and media hegemony. *Animal Studies Journal* 4, 99-125.

Perel, P et al. (2007) Comparison of treatment effects between animal experiments and clinical trials: systematic review. *British Medical Journal* 334:197; doi.org/10.1136/bmj.39048.407928.BE.

Peters, A. (2016) Liberté, egalité, animalité: Human-animal comparisons in law. *Transnational Environmental Law* 5:25-53.

Pettersson, IC et al. (2016) Factors affecting ranging behaviour in commercial free-range hens. *World's Poultry Science Journal* 72:137-140.

Phillips, CJC. (2009) A review of mulesing and other methods to control flystrike (cutaneous miasis) in sheep. *Animal Welfare* 113:113-121.

Phillips, C (2016a) *Greyhound racing ban: NSW is looking at the industry from the dogs' point of view*. The Conversation. www.theconversation.com/greyhound-racing-ban-NSW-is-looking-at-the-industry-from-the-dogs-point-of-view-62197

Phillips, C. (2016b) New South Wales overturns greyhound ban: a win for the industry, but a massive loss for the dogs. *The Conversation*. www.theconversation.com/new-south-wales-overturns-greyhound-ban-a-win-for-the-industry-but-a-massive-loss-for-the-dogs-66822

Phillips, C (2016c) The welfare risks and impacts of heat stress on sheep shipped from Australia to the Middle East. *The Veterinary Journal* 218:78-85.

Phillips, C (2017) Ringling Bros circus closure shows our changing attitudes to animals in captivity. *The Conversation* 24 January 2017.

Phillips, C and Petherick, C (2015) The ethics of a co-regulatory model for farm animal welfare research. (2015) *Journal of Agricultural and Environmental Ethics* 28:127.

Phillips, C et al. (2011) An international comparison of female and male students' attitudes to the use of animals. *Animals* 1:7-26.

Plous, S (2002) Is there such a thing as prejudice towards animals? in *Understanding prejudice and discrimination*, ed S Plous, McGraw Hill.

Productivity Commission (2017) *Regulation of Australian Agriculture*. Report No 79.

Radford, M (2001) *Animal law in Britain*. Oxford University Press.

Raworth, K (2017) *Doughnut Economics*. Random House Business.

Reid, J (2012) Wrecking Macquarie Island to save it. *The Quadrant* 11 September 2012.

Read, JL et al. (2015) Toxic trojans: can feral cat predation be mitigated by making their prey poisonous? *Wildlife Research* 42:689-696.

Regan, T (1987) *The struggle for animal rights* International Society for Animal Rights.

Richards, S (1986) Drawing the life-blood of physiology: vivisection and the physiologists' dilemma, 1870-1900. *Annals of Science* 43:27-56.

Ritskes-Hoitinga, H and Wever, K (2018) All stakeholders must act decisively to fix endemic problems. *BMJ* 360:j4935.

Robins, A and Phillips, CJC (2011) International approaches to the welfare of meat chickens. *World's Poultry Science Journal* 67:351-369.

Robbins, JA et al. (2015) Stakeholder views on treating pain due to dehorning dairy calves. *Animal Welfare* 24:399-406.

Robbins, JA et al. (2016) Awareness of ag-gag laws erodes trust in farmers and increases support for animal welfare regulations. *Food Policy* 61:121-125.

Rollin, BE (1992) *Animal rights and human morality*. Prometheus Books.

Rollin, B (2006) The regulation of animal research and the emergence of animal ethics: a conceptual history. *Theoretical Medicine and Bioethics* 27:285-304.

Rollin, BE (2007) Animal research: a moral science. *EMBO Reports* 8:521-525.

Rollin, BE (2015) The inseparability of science and ethics in animal welfare. *Journal of Agricultural and Environmental Ethics* 28:759-765.

Rose, JD et al. (2014) Can fish really feel pain? *Fish and Fisheries* 15:97-133.

RSPCA Australia (2016) *The welfare of layer hens in cage and cage-free housing systems*.

Rushen, J (1991) Problems associated with the interpretation of physiological data in the assessment of animal welfare. *Applied Animal Behaviour Science* 28:381-386.

Russell, WMS and Burch, RL (1959) *The principles of humane experimental technique*. Methuen.

Ryder, RD (1989) *Animal revolution: changing attitudes towards speciesism*. Basil Blackwell.

Sandøe, P and Jensen, KK (2011) The idea of animal welfare – developments and tensions. in C Wathes et al. (eds) *ICVAE – First International Conference on Veterinary and Animal Ethics*.

Scannell, JW and Bosley, J (2016) When quality beats quantity: decision theory, drug discovery and the reproducibility crisis. *PLOS One* 11 e0147215. doi:10.1371/journal.pone.0147215.

Scannell, JW et al. (2012) Diagnosing the decline in pharmaceutical R&D efficiency. *Nature Reviews Drug Discovery* 11:191-200.

Scarborough, R and Zalcberg, J (2017) Of mice and men: why animal trial results don't always translate to humans. *The Conversation* 30 August 2017.

Sellheim, NP (2016) The legal question of morality: seal hunting and the European moral standard. *Social & Legal Studies* 25:141-161.

Senate Select Committee on Animal Welfare (1990) *Intensive Livestock Production*.

Shaban RZ et al. (2014) *Surveillance and reporting of antimicrobial resistance and antibiotic usage in animals and agriculture in Australia*. (a report commissioned by the Department of Agriculture) - at http://www.agriculture.gov.au/SiteCollectionDocuments/animal-plant/animal-health/amria.pdf.

Sharman, K (2006) Opening the laboratory door: national and international legal responsibilities for the use of animals in scientific research-an Australian perspective. *Journal of Animal Law* 2:67-75.

Sharp, TM and McLeod SR (2016) Kangaroo harvesters and the euthanasia of orphaned young-at-foot: applying the theory of planned behaviour to an animal welfare issue. *Animal Welfare* 25:39-54.

Sherwin, CM et al. (2010) Comparison of the welfare of layer hens in 4 housing systems in the UK. *British Poultry Science* 51:488-499.

Sinclair, M et al (2016) Behavioral and physiological responses of calves to marshalling and roping in a simulated rodeo event. *Animals* 6, 30: doi:10.3390/ani6050030.

Singer, P (1975) *Animal Liberation*. Random House.

Singer, P (2000) *Writings on an ethical life*. Fourth Estate.

Smolin, LA and Grosvenor, MB (2013) *Nutrition: science and applications*. John Wiley & Sons Inc.

Sneddon, J and Rollin, B (2010) Mulesing and animal ethics. *Journal of Agricultural and Environmental Ethics* 23:371-386.

Southwell, A et al (2006) Attitudes towards animal welfare. A report prepared for the Department of Agriculture, Fisheries and Forestry. www.australiananimalwelfare.com.au/app/webroot/files/upload/files/90248%20Report%20Final%20-%20PRINT.pdf

Springer, K (2016) Methodology and challenges of a complex multi-species eradication in the sub-Antarctic and immediate effects of invasive species removal. *New Zealand Journal of Ecology* 40:273-278.

Springmann, M (2016) Analysis and valuation of the health and climate change cobenefits of dietary change. *Proceedings of the National Academy of Sciences* 113:4146-4151.

Stafford, KJ and Mellor, DJ (2011) Addressing the pain associated with disbudding and dehorning in cattle. *Applied Animal Behaviour Science* 135:226-231.

Stilwell, G et al. (2009) Effect of caustic paste disbudding, using local anaesthesia with and without analgesia, on behaviour and cortisol of calves. *Applied Animal Behaviour Science* 116:35-44.

Stilwell, G et al. (2008) Comparing plasma cortisol and behaviour of calves dehorned with caustic paste after non-steroidal-anti-inflammatory analgesia *Livestock Science* 119: 63-69.

Sullivan, R, Amos, N and van de Weerd, H (2017) Corporate reporting on farm animal welfare: an evaluation of global food companies' discourse and disclosures on farm animal welfare. *Animals* 7, 17; doi:10.3390/ani7030017.

Sutherland, MA et al. (2017) The effect of age and method of gas delivery on carbon dioxide euthanasia of pigs. *Animal Welfare* 26:293-299.

Swart, JAA and Keulartz, J (2011) Wild animals in our backyard. A contextual approach to the intrinsic value of animals. *Acta Biotheretica* 59:185-200.

Szucs, E et al. (2012) Animal welfare in different human cultures, traditions and religious faithers. *Asian-Australasian Journal of Animal Science* 25:1499-1506.

Tang, AL (2010) Calcium adsorption in Australian osteopenic post-menopausal women: an acute comparative study of fortified soymilk to cows' milk *Asia Pacific Journal of Clinical Nutrition* 19:243-249.

Taylor, N and Signal, TD (2009) Willingness to pay: Australian consumers and 'on the farm' welfare. *Journal of Applied Animal Welfare Science* 12:345-359.

Terlouw, C et al (2016) Consciousness, unconsciousness and death in the context of slaughter. Part 1. Neurobiological mechanisms underlying stunning and killing. *Meat Science* 118:133-146.

Thiriet, D (2009) Recreational hunting – regulation and animal welfare concerns. In *Animal law in Australasia*, eds P Sankoff and S White, Federation Press.

Thompson, S et al. (2007) Livestock welfare product claims: the emerging social context. *Journal of Animal Science* 85:2354-2360.

Thomson, PC et al (2014) Number, causes and destinations of horses leaving the Australian thoroughbred and standardbred racing industries. *Australian Veterinary Journal* 92:303-311.

Timoshanko, AC (2015) Limitations of the market-based approach to the regulation of farm animal welfare. *UNSW Law Journal* 38:514-543.

Tischler, J (1977) Rights for nonhuman animals: a guardianship model for dogs and cats. *San Diego Law Review* 14:484-507.

Tuomisto, HL and Joost Teixeira De Mattos, M (2011) Environmental impacts of cultured meat production. *Environmental Science and Technology* 45:6117-6123.

Twigg, LE and Parker, RW (2010). Is sodium fluoroacetate (1080) a humane poison? The influence of mode of action, physiological effects, and target specificity. *Animal Welfare* 19:249-263.

Twine, R (2017) Negotiating social relationships in the transition to vegan eating practices. In *Meat Culture* ed. A Potts; Brill.

Urquiza-Haas, EG et al. (2015) The mind behind anthropomorphic thinking: attribution of mental states to other species. *Animal Behaviour* 109:167-176.

Vapnek, J and Chapman, M (2010) Legislative and regulatory options for animal welfare. *Food and Agriculture Organisation of the United Nations Legislative Study* 104.

Vickers, KJ et al. (2005) Calf response to caustic paste and hot-iron dehorning using sedation with and without local anaesthetic. *Journal of Dairy Science*. 88: 1454-1459.

Walker-Munro, B (2015) *Cattle v The Crown*: is there a place for the Commonwealth as animal welfare guardian? *University of Queensland Law Journal* 34:363-391.

Wallach, AD et al. (2017) Cattle mortality on a predator-friendly station in central Australia. *Journal of Mammalogy* 98:45-52.

Watson, D. (2014) *The Bush*. Penguin Australia.

Watson, JB (1913) Psychology as the behaviorist views it. *Psychological Review* 20:158-177.

Watt, Y (2017) Down on the farm: why do artists avoid 'farm' animals as subject matter? in *Meat Culture*, ed. A Potts; Brill.

Weary, DM et al. (2016) Societal views and animal welfare science: understanding why the modified cage may fail and other stories. *Animal* 10:309-317.

Weber, R et al. (2007) Piglet mortality on farms using farrowing systems with or without crates. Animal Welfare 16:277-279.

Webster, AJF (1994) Meat and right: the ethical dilemma. *Proceedings of the Nutrition Society* 53:263-270.

Webster, J (2005) *Animal welfare: limping towards Eden*. Blackwell Publishing.

Webster, J (2016) Animal welfare: freedoms, dominions and 'a life worth living'. *Animals* 6:35; doi:10.3390/ani6060035.

Wein, Y et al. (2017) Avoiding handling-induced stress in poultry: use of uniform parameters to accurately determine physiological stress. *Poultry Science* 96:65-73.

Wemelsfelder, F et al. (2000) The spontaneous qualitative assessment of behavioural expression in pigs: first explorations of a novel methodology for integrative animal welfare assessment. *Applied Animal Behaviour Science* 67:193-215.

Westbury, HR et al. (2011) Extending empathy research towards animals. In *Psychology of empathy*, ed DS Scapaletti, Nova Science Publishers.

White, S (2013) Into the void: international law and the protection of animal welfare. *Global Policy* 4:391-398.

White, S (2016) Standards and standard-setting in companion animal protection. *Sydney Law Review* 38:463-490.

Wilkins, AB et al. (2015) Factors affecting the human attribution of emotions towards animals. *Anthrozoos* 28:357-369.

Williams, M (2011) Productivity shortfalls in drug discovery: contributions from the preclinical sciences? *Journal of Pharmacology and Experimental Therapeutics* 336:3-8.

Wilson, DAH (2015) *The welfare of performing animals. A historical perspective*. Springer.

Wilson, MS and Peden, E (2015) Aggression and hunting attitudes. *Society and Animals* 23:2-23.

Windsor, PA et al. (2016). Progress in pain management to improve small ruminant farm welfare. *Small Ruminant Research* 142: 55-57.

Wood-Gush, DGM et al. (1990) Behaviour of pigs in a novel semi-natural environment. *Biology of Behaviour* 15:62-73.

Woods, A (2011) From cruelty to welfare: the emergence of farm animal welfare in Britain, 1964-71. *Endeavour* 36:14-22.

Wurbel, H (2009) Ethology applied to animal ethics. *Applied Animal Behaviour Science* 118:118-127.

Zhao, Y et al. (2005) Calcium bioavailability of calcium carbonate fortified soymilk is equivalent to cows' milk in young women. *The Journal of Nutrition* 135:2379-2382